Raising Today's Baby
Second Edition

Melanie J. Wilhelm DNP, CPNP

Doctor of Nursing Practice

Certified Pediatric Nurse Practitioner

Raising Today's Baby

Second Edition

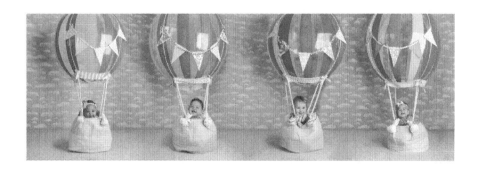

A complete guide for parenting infants birth through one year

Melanie J. Wilhelm DNP, CPNP

Doctor of Nursing Practice

Certified Pediatric Nurse Practitioner

Raising Today's Baby

Photographs in this book were provided by Leah Nisbet, Journey Through Life Photography

Copyright © 2018 Dr. Melanie J Wilhelm DNP CPNP
All rights reserved.

ISBN 10: 1725619377
ISBN 13: 978-1725619371
Raising Today's Child, Chesapeake, VA

Raising Today's Baby

This book is dedicated to my mother, Estella Frost.

She passed away June 30, 2015.

She was an amazing mother.

I was blessed to be her ladybug.

May she rest in peace.

Raising Today's Baby

Raising Today's Baby

Preface

You've all seen the pictures in magazines, and the commercials on TV: new parents welcome a beautiful baby into their household and all is peaceful and perfect. Or is it?

As a mom and a medical professional, I have found that this is a myth; that the pressure to live up to this fantasy can usher in considerable anxiety for families who expect a smooth road. A new baby causes chaos and stress, no matter how wanted, loved, or planned. Even very well read and seemingly prepared parents may be relatively inexperienced in the actual LIVE baby department. I see it every day in the office: two exhausted new parents, the mother freshly wiped out from delivery, the father exhausted from lack of sleep, and both, frankly, scared out of their minds. Rest assured, it's NOT just you. Most parents go through this stage and live to tell about it. It is NORMAL, and a few SIMPLE pointers will help. Now, take a deep breath, and read on.

Some of us live far enough away from our parents that we do not have the luxury of shared advice of past generations regarding childrearing. During the early 1900s, several generations often lived in one house, supporting and relying upon each other. This is, generally speaking, no longer the case. Today's parents may be on their own, perhaps hundreds of miles from their own parents. Even if relatives are near, their recommendations may be outdated. I know this was true in my experience. I was a military wife, 700 miles away from my home, with a new baby and a deployed husband.

Babies don't come with manuals, but parents are eager for some assistance. I know I was. They need to know what is normal and what isn't. They need to know when to worry and when to wait. They need some help; we all do. Hopefully, this book will provide that much needed assistance. And, much more.

The other books on this subject tend to be too long and too exhaustive for today's parent, who, let's face it, is pressed for time. There really is no "Dr. Spock" of our generation, advising us on all-things early parenting. There are so many different sources that you just don't know whom to trust. There are crazy conspiracy theorists, and those who alter from the recommended medical advice. You can rest assured that the views presented in this text are those of a common-sense approach to parenting. In these pages, I am replying to what my patients often ask me in the office: "Why don't you put all of this information in a book?"

I feel that this is my mission in life: to help families raise healthy, happy children. While walking on a beach, I turned to see my footsteps being washed away. I heard, "You've got to leave a deeper mark." I knew that I was being called to this mission. So, I started my journey toward this book. Learn more at www.RaisingTodaysChild.com.

I was thrilled to publish Raising Today's Baby in 2015, however, over time research yields new evidence, so an update was necessary. I hope that you will find the 2nd edition helpful and current! This includes a change not only in lay-out, but in content reflecting the current recommendations. Be sure to read the section on introducing peanut-containing foods.

These recommendations are general in nature and should not replace the advice of your healthcare provider, as the practices of medicine, parenting, and healthcare can change/evolve over time. Always seek the care of your pediatric healthcare professional.

Disclosure:

The recommendations in this book are not intended to replace regular advice from your healthcare provider. The author advocates regular medical check-ups and following the medical recommendations of your healthcare provider. The author does not assume any responsibility for any actions taken on the part of the parent. Medical recommendations change quickly. This book reflects the current information available, but always consult your pediatric healthcare provider for up-to-date information and advice.

Special thanks to:

- my husband, editor and love: Matthew Wilhelm for your support
- my kids: Brandon and Ashley-Kate, who allowed me to write about them and assisted me with tech support and website development
- my sister: Mary Ann Frost, PhD, www.MyPowerfulJourneys.com
- my photographer: Leah Nisbit, Journey through Life Photography
- my friends: Cindy & Joe O'Neil, Marg & Norm Bishop & Ann Gaine
- my mentors: Ann Roach, Ronald Ballance, Carolyn Rutledge PhD, Kathie Zimbro PhD and Laurel Garzon, PhD
- my medical editors and colleagues, who fact checked and challenged me: Robert Fink MD, Patrick Gerbus, MD, Liz Gerdun-Ashby PNP, Uyen Le-Jenkins DNP, CPNP, Leah Rowland, MD, Scott Vergano, MD, and Kelly Wright, MD
- my financial planner at Ameriprise: Albert Sganga
- my logo designer: Michael Tompkins, artist
- my spiritual leaders: Fr. Brian Rafferty, Joyce Meyer and Joel Osteen
- my trainer: Coach Early Beckwith Jr
- my personal assistant: Jennifer Williams
- my editor: Benee Knauer

Raising Today's Baby

Raising Today's Baby

Table of Contents

Chapter 1:   Parent questions

Chapter 2:   Finding balance as a parent

Chapter 3:   Sleep…or the lack thereof

Chapter 4:   Why are they still crying?

Chapter 5:   Bath time and bubbles

Chapter 6:   Medical care 411

Chapter 7:   Feeding time again?

Chapter 8:   Diaper duty

Chapter 9:   Working out working

Raising Today's Baby

Chapter 1: Parent questions

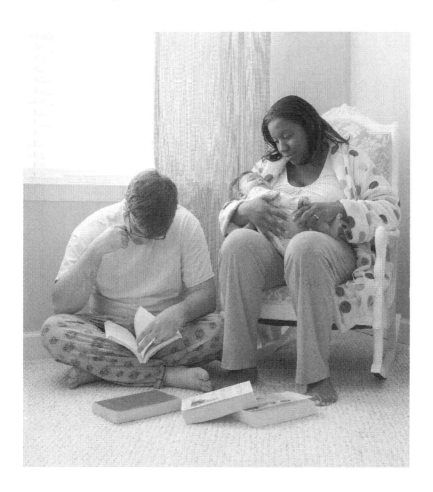

Raising Today's Baby

Chapter 1: Parent questions

As a Doctor of Nursing Practice (DNP) and a Certified Pediatric Nurse Practitioner (CPNP), I receive many questions from parents every day. Sharing their questions and my responses may be helpful to some readers. Remember, this is not a substitute for regular medical care. Always check with your pediatric healthcare provider regarding your own child. Also, know that answers change with time, as more knowledge is gained through research.

What's the best formula?

Well, we all know breast is best. Unfortunately, there are times when breastfeeding isn't possible or practical. In those cases, it is safe and effective to use an infant formula. There are several brands: Enfamil products, Similac products, and Gerber products, as well as several store brands. The categories of formula include milk-based, soy-based or specialty formulas. Most infants thrive on milk-based formulas. Brand is less important that the category of formula. If your child needs a formula change it should be recommended by your pediatric healthcare provider. Start with Enfamil Infant or Newborn, Similac Advance, or Gerber Good

Start (all are milk-based), or you can choose a store brand formula which is equivalent at half the price of brand name formulas (please see Chapter 7). Gerber Good Start Gentle formula add probiotics to support gut health. My children both thrived on Similac products.

At what age should I start disciplining my child?

That question sounds a little scary to me. Babies don't need discipline; they need love and care. If a baby is crying, it is because they are expressing a need. Crying is an infant's only language. Now, agreed, at a certain age most children become mischievous and get into things. Usually that isn't until they are walking well, which is well over a year. Until that time, I do not recommend discipline. If they are crawling toward a danger, I would recommend moving the child or the dangerous item. My next question is why are they being allowed to crawl in a dangerous area? Baby-proofing should help. Also, knowing your child's limitations and having reasonable expectations is vital to understanding a child's behavior. Sometimes it's just nap time, for both parents and baby. It's unreasonable to expect a baby to handle a full day mall shopping trip without melting down. Movies also are bad ideas, as are fancy quiet restaurants. Set realistic goals and expectations. Time-outs are for children over a year and should not exceed one minute per year of life (a two-year-old gets a two-minute time out). This will be covered more extensively in: *Raising Today's Toddler*, available soon on Amazon!

How do you feel about cloth diapers?

I think cloth diapers are a great friend to the environment. Having said that, I used them for about a half a minute before I gave up. Today's cloth diapers are much friendlier, with snaps rather than pins. There can be an increased risk of diaper rash with cloth, as they don't keep the skin quite as dry as disposable diapers do, but with vigilant changing and an effective diaper cream, they work just fine. If you don't mind the laundry (or you have a service), cloth diapers are a significant cost savings and a great gift to our world environment. You do need to consider the cost of water and electricity to launder the diapers as well. Chapter 8 has more information on diapers.

What's your favorite diaper cream?

That's easy…I have two. My favorite is Vitamin A+D ointment. I like it because it's a great barrier cream to protect the skin, but also because it is clear, so that you can see the skin. My second favorite is any cream with

Zinc Oxide (Desitin and Butt Paste are both good). Zinc oxide is good for open sores in the diaper area. These raw areas won't hold some creams, but the zinc gets in there and sticks to protect the raw area and to allow for healing. If you don't have either, Vaseline takes a close third. You can put Vaseline almost anywhere. It's good for the diaper area, also helpful for chapped hands, lips, or cheeks. Vaseline works great when applied on top of lotion on dry baby skin…wait can I change my answer to Vaseline??? Read more about skin care in Chapter 5.

What soaps and lotions do you recommend?

I recommend Johnson & Johnson head to toe or Dove unscented soap. I recommend many lotions, all of which are dye-free and fragrance-free, including Aveeno, Lubriderm, or Cetaphil. Stay away from the fragranced soaps and lotions. Even lavender, which is all natural, can be irritating to baby's delicate skin. Look for sensitive skin products. Chapter 5 discusses bathing and skin care in more detail.

How often should I burp my baby?

A baby should be burped at least after every feeding, but sometimes I will burp in the middle of the feed as well. I don't recommend the middle of the feed burp for every child, as some babies will not go back to the bottle or breast after being burped. More important than how often should you burp, is your technique of burping. A burp should be firm with a cupped hand, with sufficient force to get a burp, but not too hard to leave a mark or shake the baby. Never shake a baby, as it can cause brain damage or even death. See Chapter 7 on feeding for more information on burping.

Is it possible to both breastfeed and bottle feed?

Not only is it possible, but many parents do both. If you are breastfeeding and you wish to introduce the bottle, I recommend you introduce the bottle early, generally before six weeks of age, and offer at least one bottle every day, so it becomes a normal habit. This may make it easier for your breast-fed infant to accept the bottle. If you plan to return to work, consider starting a daily bottle before six weeks of age. When you introduce formula, you may notice a change in the infant's stool. Formula produces a much more formed stool, and you may notice fewer bowel movements with formula. Chapter 7 on feeding will give you further details. Remember a baby's stool normally changes in frequency around two months of age as well. Look into this topic in Chapter 8 diaper duty.

What can I do if my baby won't sleep through the night?

Well, you are talking to the queen of *my child won't sleep through the night*. My daughter was three years old before that happened. I feel like it's something you can encourage, but can't force. (You can lead a horse to water, but you can't make him drink.) Until the magic happens, try feeding in shifts. I would feed at 9 p.m., then sleep from 9 p.m. to 3 a.m., then I'd wake for the 3 a.m. feeding. My husband would stay up to do the midnight feed, then he slept from midnight to 6 a.m. We both got at least six hours, which in our case was the bare minimum we needed for survival and normal functioning. We weren't well rested, but we did make it. You can also stop night time feedings between six and nine months (with your pediatric healthcare provider's blessing and supervision if your child is growing well), which may help your child to sleep through the night. Speak to your provider to be sure that your child has enough weight gain to stop nighttime feedings before you do so. Hang in there! Eventually, they go to college, where they don't sleep through the night either, but finally you can. Chapter 3 discusses sleeping further.

What's the best age to return to work?

That's a personal question, and certainly depends upon your situation. I like to encourage folks to take 12 weeks of maternity/paternity leave if they can. In a perfect world, it would be great if the babies could be home until they have had two sets of immunizations (four months of age) to protect them from disease. Personally, I found life got overall easier after my children turned six months. Perhaps it took me that long to get into the rhythm of infant care. Trust me, it does get easier. Please refer to Chapter 9 on working for more discussion.

How do you feel about co-sleeping?

The American Academy of Pediatrics discourages co-sleeping due to the risks of suffocation, falls, and accidental deaths which can occur. Some folks have rolled over and crushed their tiny infant. A friend just shared that this happened to someone she knew. Babies can suffocate in the loose soft bedding. It's not worth the risk. I do not recommend it for you or for my patients, but I realize that in many countries it is done. Many of those countries do not have the very soft bedding which we have in America. Be warned that it can be a fatal mistake due to suffocation risks. Safety first. This is so not worth the risk. Infants should sleep in their parent's room, but on a separate sleep surface such as a crib. Read more in Chapter 3: Sleep...or the lack thereof.

Is it important to do the well-baby checks?

It is vital to do your well-baby check-ups. It is during these visits that we find many issues that can affect your child's overall health and development. You should plan for a well visit around 24 to 48 hours after leaving the hospital, then several times in the first two weeks. After that it's done routinely at two weeks, 2, 4, 6, 9, 12, 15, 18 months and 2, 2 ½, and 3 years and yearly after that. If you aren't sure if your child is due for their next well check-up, call your pediatric office and ask. I usually recommend scheduling your next well visit when you leave the office. I can't tell you how many serious problems I have found on well exams. It's good to find problems early so that we can give the appropriate medical care for the problem. You can find more information about check-ups in Chapter 6: Medical care.

What if I'm not sure about vaccines?

Your pediatric healthcare provider should be someone you trust. It is their honor and privilege to help you care for and protect the health of your child. They should help you understand vaccines and explain that vaccines are safe and effective. It is far riskier for you to put your child in a car than to give your child a vaccine. Still, if you have specific questions and concerns, they can provide evidence-based answers (based on research). Facts are more important than fear. Always ask to see the VIS (Vaccine Information Sheet) which explains what each vaccine is for, who should take it, when it is given and any normal side effects which can occur. Your provider should take the time to explain how vaccines work, as well as what the disease can do. Many people don't know that the vaccines protect against life-threatening diseases that can kill babies. After reviewing the VIS, you may feel more comfortable about your child receiving vaccines. Why wouldn't we want to protect our precious babies from these terrible diseases? I once had a grandmother at a picnic tell me about how she lost a grandchild to a vaccine preventable disease. She made me promise that I would tell parents that they can prevent these unnecessary deaths just by getting their children vaccinated. Please refer to Chapter 6: Medical care for more information on vaccines.

If my baby is large (high percentile), and seems unsatisfied, can I start introducing food?

Regardless of your child's size, food should not be introduced until at least four months of age. If you have a family history of food allergies, the introduction of food should be delayed until closer to six months of age. If your large baby seems unsatisfied, you can increase the amount or frequency of formula or breast milk. I always want a baby to be satisfied after a feeding. Chapter 7 on feeding can give you more details.

Is it okay to add cereal to the bottle?

Overall, babies need to eat with spoons, so I generally recommend offering the cereal with a spoon and not in a bottle. Cereal, since it's a food, should not be introduced until at least four months. There are times in my clinical practice when I break that rule. If I have a baby with bad reflux (spitting up), I sometimes will trial adding cereal to the bottle to help the formula stay down. There are formulas that already contain cereal, such as Enfamil AR or Similac for Spit-Up. Speak to your healthcare provider before adding cereal to your child's bottle or before changing your child's formula. If you are adding cereal such as oatmeal as part of your child's diet, do so using a spoon after four to six-months of age. Please see Chapter 7 on feeding for more information.

Should I give my baby a bath if he/she is sick and has fever?

Bathing is generally not harmful for minor illnesses like colds. You want the water to be comfortable and warm. You don't want the baby to get chilled, so drying quickly is important. If a child has a fever (temperature greater than 100.4 degrees F), I would recommend Tylenol. If the Tylenol doesn't seem to be bringing down the temperature a warm bath can do so. You don't want to put a feverish child in a cool bath, as it may produce a too rapid temperature change, but a warm bath would be fine. Seek medical care if your child is ill. There's more discussion about illness in Chapter 6: Medical care.

At what point (fever-wise) do I head to the Emergency Room (ER)?

This is a great opportunity for me to discuss the fear of fever. Fever is feared and dreaded by parents, but fever is really a friend. It tells us when our child is ill. It helps kill the germs that are making the child ill. Fever is not to be feared, but respected. Any temperature over 100.4 degrees F in an infant under two months old, warrants a visit to the Emergency Room. If your child has a fever, I would recommend you contact your pediatric healthcare provider, or the nurse line. Fever is only one aspect of the picture. We need to consider how the baby is acting, sleeping, and eating. We need to know how long the baby has been sick. Generally, children can safely run temperatures up to 104 degrees F. If your child's fever is higher than 104 degrees F, then call your provider or seek medical care. If you child (over two months old) has a temperature of greater than 100.4 degrees F for more than three days, they should be evaluated in your pediatric office. **ANY** fever in an infant less than two months old calls for an immediate trip to the emergency room. I try to save the emergency room visits for things like seizures and head injuries, however, if you call your after-hours pediatric provider and they direct you to the emergency room, then it's time to go. Learn more in Chapter 6: Medical care 411.

What is your take on antibiotics?

In my opinion, antibiotics are the miracle of our century. Antibiotics kill bacterial infections. They do not work on viruses (like colds or flu). They have saved more lives than I can even imagine. When my mother was a child, people died of simple infections. After my mother lost her first child (full term) due to sepsis (infection), she waited to die. The baby had died just days before delivery. They left her abdomen open so that the pus and infection could escape. They came around with the "new medicine" Sulfa (an antibiotic) and sprinkled it directly into her open gaping abdominal wound. Each day, the nurses would lay gauze to soak up the pus and infection. Slowly, she recovered. I have no doubt that my mother would not have lived if it were not for the discovery of antibiotics, and I would have never been born.

Having said that, the concern of today is the over-use and misuse of antibiotics, which has led to antibiotic resistance. Germs are smart. They change. They overcome their obstacles. Their obstacles include antibiotics.

Antibiotics are safe and effective when used appropriately and diligently. They should not be prescribed haphazardly. If your healthcare provider feels your child needs antibiotics, I do feel you should gladly take them. I do not feel you should demand them for every viral illness your child has, as they don't work for viruses.

Should I worry about over-prescribed medications?

The literature states that healthcare providers are doing a better job of NOT over prescribing antibiotics. I think both parents and providers understand that antibiotics must be used judiciously, and only as needed. If your healthcare provider recommends an antibiotic, it's fine to ask why. I never mind explaining why it's important to treat bacterial infections with antibiotics. Antibiotics kill the bacteria causing certain infections, such as urinary tract infections.

I still worry about medications which should NOT be given to children. There is a recommendation that children under the age of four years receive NO cough or cold medications, as they are not safe for children. Babies less than a year should receive no medication other than what is recommended by your healthcare provider, which may include infant Tylenol.

What about side effects of medications?

All medications have side effects. There's a well-known story about a class of medical students who are given a handout to read about potential side effects of a medication. The side effects include risk of severe skin reaction, anaphylaxis, hepatotoxicity (liver toxicity), nephropathy (kidney disease), anemia, nausea, rash, and headache. The list went on and on. The students were asked if they would take the medicine. Most said no way! Then they told the medical students that the medication was Tylenol. You can imagine their shock. This demonstrates that even one of the "mildest" medications does indeed have side-effects. Still, it is safe and effective to use, even in infants at the correct doses.

Medications for babies are dosed based on weight and not age. Side effects of antibiotics include loose stools, diaper rash, and nausea. Taking antibiotics with food or formula can minimize those effects. I also recommend a children's probiotic to help put back the good bacteria in the gut when giving antibiotics.

What do you suggest if my baby will only take an ounce during over-night feedings and then wakes again an hour later for more? Is there a way to get the baby to eat more in a single feeding?

A newborn normally only takes one to one and a half ounces per feeding, so that would be a normal amount if you have a new baby. Older babies tend to increase their feeds, but most babies need to feed about every three hours. I do not recommend feeding every hour. Even with newborns, I recommend feeding no more often than every two and a half hours. Breast-fed babies tend to snack more but will adhere to a schedule once it's established. I don't know of a way to make your child drink more, but I would certainly check the drip rate of the nipple. If the child must work too hard to get milk, they get tired before they get much out. A bottle should drip freely if turned over. If your bottle doesn't drip, place a larger hole in the nipple with a clean scissor or a needle (heated with flame). The bottle should drip like a leaky faucet. Also, if a child is fed every hour, they are not very hungry and may be crying because their stomach hurts from a too frequent feeding schedule. Give the baby a pacifier and wait for at least three hours between feedings. I like to keep babies on a schedule to help me know when the next feeding will be (6:00, 9:00, 12:00, 3:00, 6:00). Most babies can finish a bottle or feeding within 20 to 30 minutes.

At what point, if milestones are missed, should I worry and consult the pediatrician?

We check for developmental milestones at every well examination (ages 2, 4, 6, 9, 12, 15, 18, 24, 30, and 36 months). If at any point you notice a delay, please discuss this with your pediatrician. It is better to evaluate these issues sooner rather than later. If special services are needed, such as physical therapy or speech therapy, the sooner we begin, the better. If I notice a delay, I will point it out to the parent and tell them I'm concerned. We often watch delays for a couple of months, as most children will catch up by the next visit. For example, some children are not rolling by four months, but at the six month visit they roll like crazy. If they are still not rolling at six months, then it may be time to evaluate. We may have them see a specialist or receive physical therapy. Other therapies can be ordered for delayed language or behavior, including speech therapy or occupational therapy.

What do you suggest if I have a concern about my baby's development, and the pediatrician says all is well? Do I reach out to a specialist?

The relationship between a parent and provider is one of mutual listening, trust and respect. I try to listen and provide sound counsel. Sometimes parents are concerned since they don't know what is normal for that age. I had parents that were concerned that their child wasn't speaking in sentences yet, but I assured them that it was a bit early for sentences. They were then reassured. It sounds to me like you were NOT reassured by your pediatric visit. In that case, I'm wondering if your concerns are indeed founded. I would first suggest you obtain a second opinion by perhaps another pediatric provider. I often offer that option to parents if they question my logic. It helps to have another head in the mix. I ask one of my colleagues to speak with the parents. You can always seek another opinion. Most insurance policies require a referral prior to seeing a specialist and there may be an extended wait to see a specialist. Seek a second opinion if needed.

How do I know when to worry about differences in the development of my two children? While they move at different paces, what are the signs to watch for that might signal problems?

It's difficult not to compare children, but I encourage parents to try. Each child is a unique and separate individual. No two children are exactly the same. Parents know their children better than anyone else. If your child has missed developmental milestones on two or more visits, some intervention is warranted. Referral to a specialist, therapy, or additional testing should be recommended. There are ranges of normal, and your pediatric healthcare provider should explain to you the ranges of normal. Perhaps four to six words are expected. Your child only has two words, "mama" and "dada." Upon further questioning, you admit the child says "uh-oh" if they drop something and "ba" for bottle. That's four words and it meets the minimum criteria. I would reassure you that your child is normal, even if your other child had 20 words at this age. If you are interested in a good text discussing children's development, get the Bright Futures text which is available on

Amazon. If you are concerned about your child's development, discuss your concerns with your pediatric provider.

How worried should I be about keeping my baby away from others with colds and other germs? What about siblings who are sick?

The less exposure babies have to people, particularly crowds, can mean the less exposure that the child has to illness. Babies, particularly young babies, have greater risk since they are not yet vaccinated. The first set of vaccines occurs at two months of age, and until that time infants should avoid crowds including malls and restaurants. Pertussis (whooping cough) is particularly worrisome in this age group, since it can be life-threatening and is present in many communities. Getting the Dtap (diptheria, tetanus, and pertussis) vaccination at two, four and six months can decrease the risk of pertussis. Siblings who are ill should be kept apart from the baby as much as possible. Teach siblings not to kiss babies on their faces or hands to decrease the spread of germs. Discourage the sharing of drinks or the placing of infant pacifiers in siblings' mouths. Kissing the back of the baby's head is much safer. I understand that we can't live in a bubble, but the less exposure the infant has, the less risk. Still, sometimes you need to get groceries.

How does getting viruses help to build my baby's immune system?

The body works by first recognizing a virus as a foreign invader, then elevating the temperature to try to kill it. It takes the body about a week to 10 days to produce antibodies to fight the virus (hence how long a cold lasts). Once the body has developed antibodies against a certain virus, then the body recognizes it the next time it is exposed and can fight it off without becoming ill. This is also how vaccines work, except instead of introducing a live disease, we introduce a dead or weakened disease to allow the body to make the antibodies. There are many viruses out there; in fact, there are as many as 200 strains of the common cold. It takes cold after cold, virus after virus for our bodies to develop the necessary antibodies, but over time we do. That's why preschoolers always have runny noses, but high schoolers rarely do.

When do I stop sterilizing nipples for bottle feedings?

Whenever you want, really. Nipple sterilization has more or less gone the way of bottle sterilization. With the invention of the dishwasher, nipples are heated highly enough to kill any bacteria. Really the only folks I encourage to boil nipples are those who wash bottles by hand, or babies who have been diagnosed with thrush (yeast infection in the mouth). Thrush looks like white patches and will be on the inside of the cheeks and gums, not just on the tongue. If you are concerned your child has thrush, see your pediatric provider, as they will need a prescription treatment, usually Nystatin suspension.

There has been some discussion in the medical community that all the cleanliness is overkill, and that we may not be doing our children a favor by sterilizing everything around them. The mouth is not a sterile environment, nor does it need to be. If you have a dishwasher, use it. If you are washing by hand, use hot water and if it makes you feel better, go ahead and boil those nipples. I sure did, probably unnecessarily, but it made me feel better. Did I mention both my children have asthma and allergies? We wonder if those diagnoses are linked to over-cleanliness…food for thought. The jury is still out.

How can I tell, from prolonged crying, if my baby is just fussy or if something is really wrong?

Boy, this question makes me nervous. It necessitates many other questions, such as is there a fever? How long has this gone on? How is the baby feeding? When was the last stool? Is the baby vomiting? At the end of the day my advice is simple, if you as the parent feel like something is wrong, trust your instinct and have your child immediately evaluated by your pediatric healthcare provider. You don't know how many parents I've been able to reassure with a simple exam. If nothing is wrong, you don't have to worry, and if something is wrong, then we need to find it and deal with it. Always seek medical care for prolonged crying. Crying is the only form of communication your baby has, and we need to find out what it means. Don't wait. Learn more in Chapter 6: Medical care.

Thank you!

Thanks to all of you whose questions over the years prompted me to write this book. If you have a question that I didn't cover, I urge you to find a pediatric provider who will listen to your questions and take the time to discuss your concerns.

Chapter 2: Finding balance as a parent

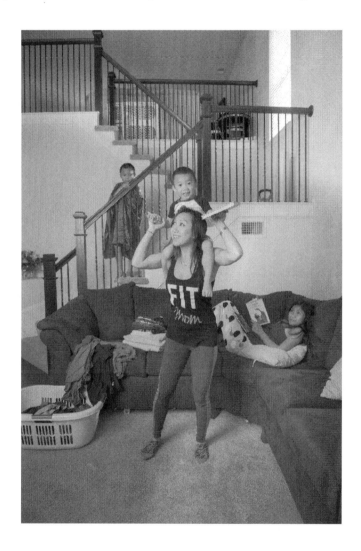

Raising Today's Baby

Chapter 2: Finding balance as a parent

As a new parent, I felt out of balance. I certainly felt like I didn't have the time or energy to consider taking care of myself, but what I didn't realize was that if I didn't care for myself, there wasn't much left for anyone else. I know you are tired; no, make that, exhausted. I remember feeling that way as well. I also remember not feeling very good about myself. Here I had just created the best thing I could in the world, a new life, and I felt out of balance myself. Looking back, it was those difficult times that lead to my life's work, helping parents and children have happy, healthy lives. Part of helping you is helping you care, not only for your child, but for yourself.

Your life is now devoted to caring for a baby; your life is forever changed. You will never again go to sleep worried about nothing. You will never again wake wondering what to do next. You will care for this child with every breath you take for the rest of your life. BUT who will care for you? As parents, we tend to be caregivers and we're great at it. We are not so great at caring for ourselves. We may need a bit of reminding that we need care as well. We need to keep ourselves and our lives in balance.

I often say, babies don't always read the books...meaning that babies may not always follow what's normally expected. Some babies talk earlier and walk later. Some don't get any teeth until after 12 months. Some cry for hours no matter what the parents try. It sometimes happens, but when it happens to you, it's important for YOU to get the support YOU need to get through the tough times. Support is needed in many areas. You must find the balance in your life as a parent. You are the only one that can take care of you. People used to say to me, "Oh take care of yourself." I used to think, sarcastically, *"Thanks a lot."* But that statement does mean something. It means that no one can care for you as an adult. Oh sure, we can help others, but only you can really choose a healthier lifestyle for yourself.

I am going to review ten areas of your life that need your attention, now more than ever. I believe that when we get out of balance in one area it affects all the others. These areas are exercise, nutrition, appearance, rest, emotional support (friendship), spiritual support (faith), health, environment, goals and recreation/hobbies. Even if you feel like you can't possibly address all these areas right now, choose one at a time and make a small improvement. Then move on to another. Our lives become our habits. As we get into healthier habits, we will have healthier lives. I really believe that healthier lives lead to happier lives. Take a deep breath now, and dig in. It may be difficult to think about all of these, but it can help you to improve in even one area.

Exercise

Let's begin with exercise. Why is it that as parents we are so in tune with what's best for our children, and yet not so in tune with what's best for ourselves? Why will we obsess over getting our kids to their baby gym dates, but we haven't seen the gym ourselves for quite some time. We don't let our kids miss even one practice, but we skimp on time to exercise ourselves. I'll be honest, I don't love to exercise. A favorite saying of mine is, "Exercise? I thought you said accessorize!" That tells you how excited I am to exercise. Honestly, it's a real chore for me. But, I know how important it is for you both physically and mentally. Exercise helps alleviate both anxiety and depression. It helps with baby weight. It helps in so many ways. I try to find fun things I like to do, like dancing, so I enjoy Zumba classes or jazzercise. I try to schedule it three times a week for 30 to 60 minutes, with a friend, so I'm less likely to back out. I also work with a professional trainer once a week who pushes me beyond my comfort zone to try to work on strength and balance. Maybe you could go for a walk with a friend. You could put the baby in a stroller and take a walk or jog. Even a walk around the mall is exercise…skip the pretzel bites. Make a date for a tennis match. Join a buddy for racquetball. Sign up for softball. Go for a bike ride. Just put on some music and dance. Cleaning can be great exercise. I sweat every time I mop the floor. My husband enjoys playing ice hockey with our son. Just move.

If you're not ready to jump into an exercise program yet, try a daily walk. This is good both for you and the baby. Walking is a great exercise and all you need is a decent pair of sneakers. Start out by walking 10 minutes out and 10 minutes back. Increase your time until you can walk for 45 minutes each day. Try to walk faster than is comfortable. You should be able to speak, but may be breathing harder than normal. I recommend that you consult with your healthcare provider prior to beginning any exercise program to determine if you are healthy enough to begin regular exercise. Exercise will help you be a better parent, as your moods will improve, you will feel better physically and emotionally. It's a good habit to model for your children. Children learn what they live. Try to add some exercise into your life, even two to three times a week, and watch for positive results. Your kids will thank you and honestly, your jeans will thank you.

Nutrition

Now, what about your nutrition? I am constantly amazed by how conscious parents are about what they feed their children, but they will eat anything that's in front of them. Many parents make their baby's food from all natural products, but are not so particular with what is going in their own mouths. Why wouldn't we as parents want to model healthy eating? The healthier we eat, the healthier our children will eat as well. You are very important in the life of your child. You need to eat wholesome nutritious foods just as they do.

I make a meal list each weekend for the week ahead. After planning my meals, I write the grocery list. This way, anyone can go to the store (as opposed to when I keep my list in my head). I start the dinner prep in the morning before work by defrosting and marinating the protein. I set out the ingredients and dishes. After a long day, I just look at the meal list and I know what's for dinner. It minimizes the thought process, so I'm less likely to order pizza or grab a burger out. Also, with everything set out ahead of time, whoever gets home first can start dinner. A bit of early planning pays off with a healthier diet, and it's less expensive than impulse dining. I set the table before I leave for work, so there's less chance we'll scrap the plan and grab fast food.

Recently, I was having some trouble with weight, so I sought the advice of a registered dietician (also called a nutritionist), who made some recommendations. First of all, she suggested that I journal my diet. Anything that went into my mouth went into the journal. If you have a smart phone, there are several free apps that can help. I like the free app "Lose It". My nutritionist recommends the free app "My Fitness Pal." After journaling what I ate normally for a week, she reviewed it. I was surprised to hear that she felt I did not consume enough protein. When I told her that I was exhausted and starved by 3 p.m. daily, she explained that my body burned quickly through the carbohydrates, but since I lacked the protein my energy was not sustained. As I balanced my diet nutritionally, not only did I shed the unwanted pounds, but I had more energy and stamina. You may be surprised to find that a meeting with a nutritionist is not very expensive. I recommend you seek out a registered dietician familiar with breastfeeding (if you are doing so). Do not cut your calories lower than is recommended by your OB/GYN. Weight Watchers is another valuable resource for learning to control one's diet and weight. Weight Watchers also has an app to track your intake and an online support group for encouragement.

Remember that a healthy diet should include the four basic food groups: meat/protein, starches/carbohydrates, fruits/vegetables and milk/cheese. Try to limit sweets and include healthy fats (olive oil). Try to eat lean meats, whole grain breads (100% whole wheat), and fresh fruits and vegetables. Remember that if you are breastfeeding, you will need to consume extra calories in order to produce milk. Don't forget to continue your prenatal vitamins. Always seek the advice of your healthcare provider before changing your diet plan. Remember that you need to have energy to care for your child. Energy comes from a healthy diet, so don't starve yourself. Why not make what you consume as important as what your baby consumes? If you eat well, you will have the energy and health to be the best parent you can be. You are the role model for your children to follow.

Appearance

How cute are baby clothes? Let's face it; any infant clothing is adorable. There's the animal wear with ears and tails, there's the girlie dresses with full skirts and matching tights…there's nothing not to like about how our babies look in their clothes. We will buy them too many outfits even though they will quickly outgrow them. But how is our appearance? Why do we spend the money to dress them up like dolls, when we look like we haven't shopped in years?

When we are exhausted from caring for a child, we tend to let ourselves go. I was guilty of this. I just didn't have the energy to do anything more than shower daily for a while (and some days I skipped that). I had to pull myself out of my formula-stained t-shirt and sweatpants (you should have seen me) and into a nice sweater and jeans. OK, so I had to wear my maternity jeans for a while after delivering. It happens. But a little makeup on the face and a flat iron to the hair can do wonders for your spirit. Sometimes you have to buy one or two outfits in a larger size until you lose the baby weight. One of my secrets is that I had some friends who would exchange clothes as we changed sizes. Another trick: try thrift stores. A well put together outfit makes you feel better no matter the size. It's not about a size or a number, it's about the look and the accessories. Maybe a chunky bangle, or a dangle earring. Just something to make your look pop. Not only will you feel brighter, but the joy of parenthood will show through in your appearance.

Put on some make-up. I believe strongly in the five minute face. From shower to door, I'm out of the house in 30 minutes. That includes hair and make-up. It doesn't take an hour to look better. I used to bring the baby seat into the bathroom and talk to my baby as I did my hair and make-up. (Please be sure not to spray hairspray or other scented products around your baby.) Feel free to chat with your baby as you get ready in the morning. Babies are surprisingly good listeners. A little foundation, a bit of shadow, a swipe of brush and some lip gloss. Stay away from dark colors and stick to a neutral pallet to minimize your time. How about some polish for your nails and toes? A professional mani/pedi may be just the trick. I see lots of moms bringing their kids with them for services. I don't recommend this as I don't want to expose the baby to any fumes from the polish or the remover. I bet Grandma or your best friend is dying for a turn to rock the baby for a few hours. Take advantage. For dads, try a new shirt, or a bright tie. Some bright socks or new shoes may do just the trick. Dads need sprucing up as well. I remember my husband's switch from the tennis shoes of his youth to adult leather shoes. Brightening your teeth may give a boost. Everyone can benefit from a little effort.

Is it time for a cut or some color? I know when my hair grows out I can't do a thing with it. It just lays flat on my head. A new "do" makes me feel like a rock star. Search around, there are reasonable salons who do a great job. Especially economical are salon schools where students practice under instructor supervision for a minimal price. Moms and Dads both need a trim from time to time. A new cut can help your appearance.

Sometimes a girl just needs a new bag. I don't mean a diaper bag. One of my favorite bags (and I do love my bags) I got on sale for $35. (Don't tell anyone.) I tied a scarf on it from the dollar tree, and am complimented on it everywhere I go. Just picking it up to head out of the house boosts my spirits. Take a look in the mirror…is there room for improvement? Do it, not for anyone else, but for yourself! As you feel better about how you look, you will feel better about yourself as a parent. Our moods affect how we interact with others, including our children. You take great care of your child's appearance. Doesn't your appearance deserve the same level of care? We put ourselves last too often, using all of our energy to care for our families. What we must realize is that in order to effectively care for our families, we must care for ourselves. Dads don't carry bags, but my husband takes pride in his back pack, his wallet, his belt, and his shoes. Accessories can improve everyone's appearance.

Rest

Are you exhausted just by reading these suggestions? Chances are you are not getting the proper amount of rest. Who can blame you as you have an infant under your roof? Babies are not conducive to good sleeping habits in parents. We worry about our children getting the proper rest. I had a friend cancel a lunch date with me, as her child needed a longer nap. That parent cared more about her child's rest and health than a social engagement. I applaud that, however, I wonder if she is as concerned about the amount of rest she is getting. Let's face it, you must learn to sleep around the baby's schedule. That means, you may need to nap during the day, go to bed earlier and deal with being woken at least once in the night. Remember to take care of your child effectively, you must rest properly. Your instinct is to care for your child, but you can't do that effectively if you are not caring for yourself. You need to eat right, take your vitamins and REST!!! This is true for both parents.

If you can't get a full night's sleep, grab an afternoon nap or split the feeding schedule so you can get a consecutive six hours. (One parent sleeps from 9 p.m. to 3 a.m., the other sleeps midnight to 6 a.m.). Go to bed earlier, and limit screen time (TV or computer) an hour before bedtime, as it can interfere with your ability to go to sleep. Limit caffeine. De-clutter your bedroom so that you can have a space to really relax without work or papers lying around. Turn off the baby monitor. Trust me, you'll hear the baby crying. You don't really need to hear the baby sighing, do you? Ask for help. Grandmas and friends love to "nap sit", or care for the baby while you catch a nap. Limit visitors, or use them to help you. Above all, get some proper rest. Here again, you will be a better parent if you care for yourself enough to get a proper amount of rest. I honestly did not feel rested until my kids were over a year old. I was in a constant state of sleep deprivation, and I was a miserable exhausted mess. I had to learn to put rest as a priority over say late night TV. Sometimes the housework can wait. If you are not so exhausted, you can get more done much quicker and more effectively. This is an area where I would encourage you to be selfish. Make sleep a priority.

Emotional support (friendship)

We all need emotional support, and get it in a variety of ways. I gain support from colleagues I work with, as well as family and friends. After having a baby, you are away from your work friends, and your family is well…family. Sometimes a parent just has to turn to a friend. It's great if you have a friend who has children, and has been through what you are going through as a parent. If you don't have one, find one. Join a mother's day out, or play group. Make some new friends. It's great just to gab and sometimes dump on one another. I never feel better than when laughing with a girlfriend. I meet a girlfriend at least once a month for lunch. We laugh and talk, and sometimes complain. It feels great to vent about the kids, the husband, and any problems. Husbands need their friends as well. It seems to help to join the guys to watch the game, or better yet, go to one. There's the neighborhood social group or a quick lunch with some buddies. There is nothing like the ear of a good friend. It's also great to have extended family around to help, as long as that relationship is healthy and supportive, great. If not, then you decide how much family you can handle. A wise psychologist and author (my sister, Mary Ann Frost, PhD) states that your life is like a paper bag. You decide what goes in and what stays out of your bag. You put the important things in first, then fill it with other aspects of your life. See her website at mypowerfuljourneys.com. Her book "Your life is like a paper bag" is available on her website as well as on Amazon. Another analogy is that items in your life are like pebbles in a jar. The big pebbles are things like work and commitments. The jar looks full, but you could still add some smaller pebbles. These smaller pebbles are things like groceries and exercise. Again, the jar looks full, but you can add some sand to take up the small cracks between pebbles. The sand may be friendships. Again, the jar looks full, but still holds added water. The water may be faith. Our lives can be full with work obligations, parenting obligations, bills, chores, but still there is room for friendship, laughter and fun. Find some room for your friends. Gain support to have the emotional energy you need to go back to round the clock feedings and diaper changes. Laughter and friendship will make you a better parent.

Recreation/hobbies

Speaking of fun…had any lately? I know fun gets put on the back burner when we are busy and overwhelmed with life and parenting (and sleep), but it is necessary. Some see fun as a waste of time, or unnecessary, but it is an important part of living a healthy and balanced life. Do you have any hobbies? If not, why not start one? I took up painting, and I'm really not very good at it. It doesn't matter to me. I like it. It's relaxing. It allows me to be creative, and I enjoy it. My son and I also took golf lessons so that we could play golf with my husband. Again, I'm terrible. (Both my son and husband are better.) Sometimes when we go play, I take a book and read from the cart. My husband appreciates that I make the effort. I hit a few balls and spend the afternoon with my guys. One of my favorite hobbies is going for a coffee with a friend. Here's the kicker, I don't even like coffee. I just like the coffee shop. I may get a tea, but what I love is to sit and talk with my friend or my husband. Starbucks anyone? I always recommend that my patient's parents have a date night…even once a month. Leave your angel with a trusted family member or friend and get out. Just a few hours will do you a world of good. Go to dinner and a movie, go bowling or for a walk. Just reconnect. Hold hands. Go for a drive. Enjoy each other's company. Find something you enjoy doing and do it. If you can't get a sitter, have a movie night at home. Sit together on the couch. Enjoy some popcorn. Single parents especially need some social time to escape. Arrange flowers, paint a picture, sketch a scene, paint a pot, join a club, try an activity…have some fun. Fun just might brighten your mood and help your overall health. Fun can make you a better parent. Believe me, you will soon be consumed with fun for your child…birthday parties, play dates, and scouts all await your time. Why not take one Saturday afternoon just for some fun for you?

I had a co-worker who became so overwhelmed with the demands on her as a working mother and fell into depression. Unfortunately she got little support from her husband around the house or with the kids. One day she did not come into work. Instead of seeking help, she attempted suicide, but was rescued and hospitalized in a psychiatric ward. After recovery, she shared that her medical bills cost more than a two week cruise to the Caribbean! Now which would you rather do? I decided then and there that an occasional date night and a yearly vacation was less expensive than a suicide attempt and hospitalization. Believe me, you are worth it. Your overall happiness and quality of life will improve if you take the time to improve it.

If you are having depression: get help!!! (Suicide hotline 1-800-273-8255). Seek mental health help immediately...especially if you are postpartum (just had a baby). Postpartum depression is common and dangerous...please see a mental health provider ASAP! There are medications and therapies that can help you. Your child needs a healthy parent, so please seek help. On the back of your insurance card you will find a 1-800 number for mental health services. Call it if you need help with depression or other issues. If you don't have insurance, call your local healthcare provider and ask them to direct you to mental health resources in your community. Above all, seek help. Looking back, I believe I had a minor case of postpartum depression with both births. I was fairly depressed emotionally and I was physically exhausted. I couldn't really see the situation very well while I was going through it. Hopefully my experiences will help you to be able to recognize if you are in a depression, and seek the help of a professional mental health provider. If you think you may be having postpartum depression, seek a mental health professional or speak with your doctor. Don't go through this alone. You are not alone. Seeking help for depression will make you a better parent. 1-800-PPD-MOMS.

Suicide hotline: 1-800-273-8255

Spiritual support (faith)

Your spiritual health should also not be neglected. I am a very spiritual person, but I do not judge you if you are not. I won't get into faith arguments, but suffice it to say that I believe strongly that faith (whatever faith you are) plays a strong role in finding balance and joy in life. I believe that when you put faith first and family a close second, your other obligations naturally fall into line. You need some kind of spiritual support, whether that is through a church, temple, or daily meditation. I always begin the day with scripture, prayer and meditation. It gives me the strength to press on through the difficulties of daily life. Prayer and meditation allow us to process our concerns and ease our anxiety. It allows us to acknowledge that there are things we are not in control of but believe that someone else is. A spiritual support group, such as a prayer group or meditation circle, allows us to share our life's struggles and victories with others of similar faith. It is a real joy to be able to share a faith base. Faith strengthens us when we are weak, encourages us to press on, and leads us to do better. Faith reminds us to think of others and to help others in need. Sometimes, just taking your mind off your own problems and helping someone else is very helpful. Faith unites families. Worshiping together joins us with our family in a way nothing else can. Consider your faith walk. Can you add a five minute prayer or meditation to your routine? Is there a faith-based group that you would love to join? Can you attend a service once a week? After having children, many people return to their faith as they feel it is important to hand down to their children. I know I did. I had fallen away from my faith during my youth. Particularly, in college, I was not very excited about faith, but it never really leaves you. As I had my son, I wanted to share my faith with him. I wanted my children to grow up with some sense of faith to walk in during their daily lives. I always tell my kids, I gave you three things no one can ever take away from you: a good education, a loving stable home environment, and a faith. I don't mind sharing that I am a practicing Catholic Christian. I was raised Brethren and taught the Bible. I try to be very respectful to people of all faiths. I believe that improving your spiritual self will improve your parenting regardless of what faith you choose.

Environment

Don't babies have the cutest rooms? We always fix them up, paint them and decorate. It's called nesting. We prepare our child's nest. With our first child, we were flat broke. I got all the baby furniture at yard sales and fixed them up. My husband and I (this means I chose the color and he did the work) painted an old dresser "big bird yellow" and it was bright. Thankfully the baby linens and accessories were provided by a kind baby shower. The baby's room was adorable. Here again, we fuss and fret over the baby's room, but what about our living space? Your home, what you place around you says something about you. Is your home bright? Is it clean? Is it organized? You don't have to spend a fortune to have a pleasant home. Start with one room. Set the timer for 10 minutes and tell yourself someone is going to stop over in 10 minutes…go…straighten up the best you can in 10 minutes. You will be amazed at what you can do in little bursts of cleaning. Keep cleaning supplies in the bathroom, so when you are in there you can spray the mirror, or wipe the counter. Try to clean up as you cook, so you don't have a huge mess. Never leave things overnight…it just gets worse in the morning. Never touch something twice…if you pick up the mail, separate it immediately into bills, junk to recycle, and cards. Put the bills in a container together, throw out the recycled paper and place anything else you need to deal with in a basket. Now your mail is not part of the clutter. Can't keep up with the daily paper, cancel it and check out the news online. I keep a basket at the bottom of the stairs for all the things I need to take upstairs at the end of the evening. Have hooks for coats and back packs by the door. Hooks work great for keys as well…no more searching for your keys. Maybe a few fresh flowers to brighten the kitchen and your mood. Some dads like to fuss over their garage spaces or man caves. Why not have a place you enjoy and can relax? It doesn't cost a thing to rearrange furniture. Both parents can benefit from a pleasant environment. Order trumps chaos.

I see so many people painting and re-carpeting to sell their home. Why wouldn't they paint and re-carpet for themselves? Why do it for the next guy but not your family? Stand at the entrance to your home and notice what the focal point is. Place something you love to see there, perhaps a favorite photo or painting or a nice ceramic piece. I love Tinker Bell, so I keep lots of Tink's in my office. It makes me smile. It inspires me to press on when I don't feel like pressing on. One of my Tink's says "Believe." One says "Let your dreams blossom. Surround yourself with happiness and your life will be happier." Dads like to keep trinkets on their desks as well to cheer them. I like to think of home as our refuge from the storms of life. No one wants a refuge that is chaotic and disorganized. If you don't believe me, watch the show "Hoarders" on TV. Five minutes into that show, and I'm straightening around me. Take some time to find the balance in your home, even if it's nothing more than cleaning out one drawer each evening.

It will pay off in peace and joy. If your home is pleasant and organized, how much better of a parent will you be? There's no more frantic searching for keys. There's a place for everything, and everything in its place. If you model organization, then your child will learn organizational skills as well. Again, balance in the home means balance in your life. I guess my Libra (the sign of the scales indicating balance) is showing. Balance is essential in life.

Goals

Goals are an important part of finding balance as a parent. What short term or long term goals have you set? I sometimes like to think of my goals as dreams. I sit and imagine if I could do anything, what would I really want to do. I imagine that I have no limits whatsoever. No limits of time or age. No limits of space or money. I imagine I can do anything in the world that I want to do. What do I think of? Swimming with dolphins. Climbing a mountain. Taking a cruise. All these things started on a list of possibilities, yet later became real for me. Let's face it, I'm a nobody. I came from farm land in Ohio, a child of uneducated working class people. My father was an orphaned child with an eighth grade education who grew up to work in a factory. (You can read the story of my father in the children's book entitled

"Hungry Jack," by Mary Ann Frost, PhD, available on Amazon or at www.mypowerfuljourneys.com). My mother was a cook in the factory. Not only was I able to escape the two possibilities that I could see as a young person: farm wife or factory laborer, but I went on to complete a Bachelors, Masters and Doctorate. My sister is a PhD psychologist and noted author. Her son also has his PhD and is a superintendent of schools in Michigan. My husband and both of my children have Bachelor degrees. Limits are imposed on us by our limited thinking. Where you come from does not determine where you are going. Dreams can become goals with some hard work and planning.

Set a goal, then work backwards to make it happen. Maybe you want to go back to school. Start at the end…you want to be a lawyer, well you need to go to law school, but before that you need a bachelors, so first you need to start with a college application and to learn about financial aid. Or you want to go back to work, so you need a job, to complete job applications, but first you need to polish your resume and work on a professional appearance. Maybe you've always dreamed of a trip, but never have the funds. First decide the location. Next decide if you'd like to cruise or fly. Research prices on line, and start saving…$100/month is $3600 in three years, enough for a nice trip. $200/month saved is $7200…now you can go to Europe or Hawaii. Giving up a few meals out each week can lead to savings that can be enjoyed later.

Maybe big goals are too much to think about right now. How about saving for a new outfit, or cute shoes? Maybe your goals need to be more practical during this season of your life. Maybe a new car is needed. I encourage people to have goals for this week, this month, this year, five years, and ten years. This week my goals include sticking to a healthy diet and exercise program so that at the end of this month I can fit into a favorite dress for a wedding I need to attend. This year I'm striving to increase my health to decrease my blood pressure medication, and feel better. Also I want to finish this book within this year. In five years, I'm striving to have my cars paid off and plan for a family vacation. I would like to have a series of parenting books to help you through many stages of parenting over the next five to ten years. I would also like to tour and give discussions on parenting, as well as providing parenting information over the web.

Having goals makes me a better parent. It teaches my children how to set goals and work to achieve them. Nothing ever comes without work and sacrifice. We are happy to sacrifice for our children. Setting and achieving goals will make you a more balanced parent. If it was easy, everyone would do it. It's not easy. It takes discipline and determination but it can be done. You can do anything you really want to do, if you are willing to sacrifice for it. You must be willing to pay the price.

Health

We worry constantly about our child's health. We schedule routine check-ups every few months for our baby. We get preventative vaccines to ward off diseases. We monitor their temperature. We take very good care of our children's health, but what about our own health? Health is one of those intangible things that you never miss until it's gone. You can have all the money in the world and not have health. Health is related to all these other areas we have discussed in this chapter.

If your life is out of balance, your health can be affected. Working too much or not resting? See how you feel. You need to cherish your health. We only get one body and it will only take just so much abuse before rebelling. Take your vitamins, eat lean meats, whole grains, and fresh fruit and vegetables. Get some exercise. Have some fun. Set some goals. All these things can affect your health. Get regular medical check-ups. See your dentist twice a year. Brush and floss twice daily. Take any prescribed medication as directed. Monitor your blood pressure. Drink eight glasses of water daily. Avoid alcohol and cigarettes. If you smoke, maybe it's time to consider quitting. It can be done. Watch your stress level. Women need routine gynecologic exams. Men also need routine medical exams.

Health is a continuum from completely healthy to very sick. Health can always be improved, but it takes some conscious thought and effort to do so. You're not just going to "get healthy" without some effort. Make the changes you need to make to get your life back into a healthy balance. You can do this. It is worth the effort. You are worth the effort. You can do this not only for your health, but to improve your quality of life and the health of your child. You see children learn what they live. If you live a healthy lifestyle, then so will your child. If not for yourself, do it for your baby. Find your healthy balance as a parent. You are your child's example of how to live and care for oneself in this world. Although they will meet many people, they will follow your example. Make it a healthy balanced example.

The ten areas we addressed in this chapter included exercise, nutrition, appearance, rest, emotional support (friendship), spiritual support (faith), health, environment, goals and recreation/hobbies. I hope that this helps you find happiness and balance as a parent. My wish is that my struggles and successes will inspire you to press on toward your personal goals. I hope that you can find joy, health, and happiness in parenting. Parenting has been my greatest accomplishment and my greatest joy.

Key points:

- Parenting can upset the balance in our lives.
- Finding balance can help us as parents.
- You need to care for yourself in order to care for others.
- Add some exercise two to three times each week.
- Eat a healthy diet: lean proteins, whole grains, fresh fruits & vegetables.
- Limit your sweets and fats.
- Improving your appearance will improve how you feel about yourself as a parent.
- Rest is vital, strive for eight hours daily. Take naps often.
- Connect with friends for emotional support.
- Include some fun. Find a hobby.
- Make time for prayer or meditation.
- Consider organizing your home environment.
- Set short term and long term goals.
- Get regular medical check-ups and care for your health.
- Suicide Hotline 1-800-273-8255

Chapter 3: Sleep...or the lack thereof

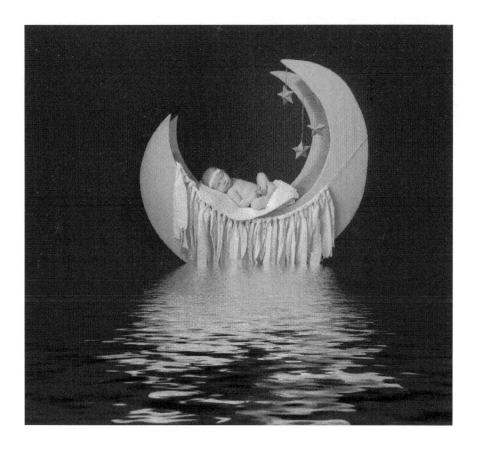

Raising Today's Baby

Chapter 3: Sleep...or the lack thereof

Babies sleep. Or do they? At least they're supposed to sleep, aren't they? Newborns do little more than wake to eat every two to three hours. In between feedings and diaper changes, they sleep blissfully while tired blurry-eyed parents stumble through the endless day-night feeding cycles. I remember this exhaustion far too well.

Sleep is an essential part of our lives. It is the time our bodies recharge and refuel. It's like plugging in your cell phone at the end of a long day. It prepares the body for the day to come. There are days I forget to charge my phone, and then I'm upset when it dies in the middle of the next day. Without sleep, we do not function at our best. Sleep impacts how we live our lives and how we feel while we do so. It impacts everything we do.

I (like you probably are now) was so tired during my children's infancies that I used to have a wish that I could sneak away and check into a hotel, alone, and just sleep until I felt rested. I probably reached this state of desperation since I had no real support system to assist me during this difficult time. My family was 700 miles away, and with my husband frequently deploying for months at a time with the US Navy, I had only myself. What I learned is that it takes a village to effectively raise a child. This is a good time to develop a support system to assist you. Joining a play group, parent's group, or church group will give you a good place to start. You could trade babysitting services with another parent, just to give yourself a break from time to time.

I remember the sheer state of exhaustion I was in during this time. Trying to drag yourself out of bed to feed a crying baby when it feels you've just fallen asleep is near to impossible. It takes every ounce of parental will you have to get up with that baby. The frustration you feel when the child will not sleep is nearly unbearable. This is where I again warn about the dangers of shaking a baby. Shaken Baby syndrome takes very little force to permanently disable or kill an infant. If you begin to feel frustrated, and it's normal that you may, put the baby in the crib on their back. Place the side rails up and take a break. Make a cup of tea and enjoy it downstairs away from the crying. Crying will not injure the baby. Shaking will. Remember shaking can kill. Never shake a baby.

Try to remember that this is a stage, and like all stages, this too shall pass. All children eventually sleep through the night. Try to keep some perspective. Although this stage is exhausting and frustrating, it is also joyous in its own right. No one else gets to spend those intimate quiet hours in the wee of the morning with your precious angel. If you ask any parent, those moments are sacred. You may not believe me right now, but you will miss them one day. You may not miss the fussiness, but you will miss watching your baby grow and develop. You will miss watching your baby coo, smile, and eventually sleep.

Sleep deprivation can cause serious issues for parents. It can affect not only their health, but their job performance, and their safety. The National Highway Traffic Safety Administration estimates that drowsy driving leads to 100,000 automobile crashes each year, causing 71,000 injuries and 1,550 fatalities. Sleep deprivation can impact your marriage or partnerships, as it impacts how you feel and act. It decreases your performance both at home and at work. Sleep deprivation can decrease not only your memory, but your ability to think and analyze problems. Overall, it affects your quality of life. Sleep deprivation also affects your health. It can lead to high blood pressure, heart disease or stroke, obesity, depression/mood disorders, and a variety of other health problems. This disruption to your body's internal clock has serious side effects. No wonder new moms often claim they have "baby brain," meaning they are not functioning at their normal levels. They are likely just sleep deprived.

It is SO true that parents need to sleep when their babies do. Try to catch a nap whenever you can – twice a day if possible! It's wonderful if your partner will split the night shift with you. One of you sleeps 9 p.m. to 3 a.m., while the other sleeps 12 midnight to 6 a.m. That way, you BOTH get at least six consecutive hours of sleep, which may not be optimal, but which will allow you to continue to function. The 9 p.m. to 3 a.m. sleeper does the 9 p.m. feed, then sleeps until the 3 a.m. feeding. The midnight to 6 a.m. sleeper stays up to do the midnight feed, but then gets to sleep through until 6 a.m. since the partner has taken the 3a.m. feed. If you can manage six hours of sleep at night, you will feel like a new person.

Most adults need between 6 to 10 hours of sleep each night. It's true that some people need more sleep than others. If we miss sleep, we need to make it up, so we'll grab a nap, or sleep in on the weekend. Baby's sleep schedule is much different from ours. They sleep more than we do, but it doesn't seem so, since their sleep cycles are divided into two to four-hour cycles.

Sleep facts

- Newborns do little more than eat, mess their diapers, and sleep. They sleep up to 17 hours each day, but usually in short one to two-hour intervals.

- Around two months of age, babies' sleep cycles tend to regulate a bit. They fall into a mid-morning and afternoon nap. They will still usually wake to feed once or twice a night but tend to have longer wakeful periods during the day. They may sleep in four or five-hour intervals at night. Their total sleep time is about 15 hours/day.

- From four to six months, the two-nap-a-day cycle will continue, but you may notice that one of the naps will get shorter (usually the morning nap). The nighttime sleep cycles continue to lengthen, thankfully. At this age, the total daily sleep time decreases to around 14 hours/day. They sleep longer at night, and less during the day.

You may notice that they even have an occasional night when they "sleep through," but then start feeding in the night again. This is usually due to growth spurts, which occur at various times. Be patient. Most babies will sleep through the night by six months, some even sooner.

> Eventually the morning nap disappears altogether. When this occurs varies but may happen in the 9 to 18-month range. Other babies may continue to be "better nappers." Children tend to take an afternoon nap until the age of three to four years, when they begin to "refuse" their nap. They chant "NO NAP" and "I'm NOT tired." Just wait and see!

What is a baby who is not sleeping be trying to tell us?

First, check the basics. Are they hungry? How long has it been since they fed? If it's longer than three hours, try offering the breast or bottle. Check the diaper; are they wet or soiled? If so, change them. Maybe they have an irritating diaper rash. Some diaper cream may soothe it. Do they need to burp? Try taking a few minutes to burp them, as this may comfort them. Rocking, swaddling, and swinging may also help. Do they seem to be in pain? Remember, crying is the infant's only language. If they cannot sleep and seem to be in pain, consult your healthcare provider immediately.

All children are different. Just because your first child was a great sleeper doesn't mean that your second child will be (or vice versa). Some babies (and adults) are just wired differently, meaning, we all have our own internal body clocks and function differently both asleep and awake. My daughter, honestly, didn't sleep through the night until she was three years old. It was a long three years. My son still sleepwalks, even as an adult. People have different sleep issues and different sleep patterns, and so do babies. Some are great sleepers, and others are tuned to a different channel. Why did my kids have to be bad sleepers? Maybe I had to live through those long nights so that I could help others with similar issues.

There has been much debate about different strategies to get babies to sleep longer. Many parents and grandparents believe that adding solid food will help children to sleep through the night. Scientific study has proven this not to be true. Remember, baby foods should not be introduced prior to the four to six-month period. Doing so may cause other issues, such as increasing the risk of food allergies and the risk of obesity.

Sleep position

Sleep positions have not changed for nearly 20 years. Sleeping on the back has been found to be the safest position. Placing a baby on his/her back to sleep decreases the risk of sudden infant death syndrome (SIDS), previously known as "crib death." I do not recommend placing infants on their stomachs or sides, unless they are awake and supervised, and then only for play time in small intervals. It is safe to do **awake** tummy time for 15 to 20 minutes two to three times each day, but the child should be supervised on a firm, safe surface where they cannot fall.

Some babies do seem to prefer to sleep on their stomachs. I know that this can be a difficult situation, but it is so much safer to sleep them on their backs that I continue to encourage parents to keep trying. Eventually, most babies will accept a back-sleeping position as normal if we keep laying them in that position while full, dry, and drowsy. There should be no bumper pads, wedges, stuffed animals, pillows, or other objects in the infant's crib.

There should be a firm mattress in the crib. I recommend using a warm fuzzy sleeper or sleep sack to eliminate the need for a blanket.

Swaddling

If you prefer to use a blanket, infants less than two months can be swaddled in a receiving blanket to keep them comfortable. Do not over-dress your child. Swaddling is done by wrapping a receiving blanket firmly around the infant, then placing them on their back. I usually put the infant's head on one corner, then wrap the opposite corner up on their feet, securing it all by wrapping the sides. It's a bit like making a burrito. It makes babies feel safe to be snuggled in their blanket. It reminds them of the womb. They sleep well when they are warm, secure, full, burped, and dry. There is an increased risk of Sudden Infant Death Syndrome (SIDS) with swaddling IF the child is placed on their stomach. Babies should ALWAYS sleep on their backs to decrease the risk of SIDS. Also swaddling too tightly can cause hip problems (hip dysplasia) so swaddle in a hip-healthy manner which allows the baby's legs to bend up and out. The hips need to able to move. A sleep sack or fuzzy sleeper works perfectly and eliminates the need for a blanket.

Co-sleeping

Co-sleeping is something of a controversial subject. Many people in other countries co-sleep with their infants. The bedding situation in other nations is somewhat different from what we are accustomed to in the USA. In developing countries, these folks may be sleeping on hard floors or on a mat. In the United States, we tend to have very soft mattresses. I do not recommend co-sleeping with your baby, as it increases the risk of suffocation for the infant. It is simply not safe. Having said that, I understand how easy it is to fall asleep with your infant in your arms while you are in bed. You are exhausted. If you are breastfeeding, it's so tempting just to bring that baby to your bed to nurse. You are relaxed, and you can easily drift off. But what if you roll over? A baby can easily suffocate with a body next to them, and in soft bedding. It's just not a safe decision. I recommend you get up, sit in a chair to nurse, and then put the baby back into the crib or basinet. You should keep the crib or basinet in your room, at least for the first few months. The American Academy of Pediatrics recommends that infants sleep on their back in the same room as their parents, but on a separate surface (crib or bassinet) for at least six months and preferably one year. A basinet is fine for most small babies up to about two to four months. After that time, the baby becomes more active and should be sleeping in a crib with the side rails up. Once you understand that the risk of co-sleeping is suffocation and potential death, I'm sure you will agree that no amount of convenience is worth your child's life. Even though you may feel absolutely exhausted you will pull yourself up, drag yourself out of bed, and feed that baby. I understand if you have a few exhausted tears during the night. I sure did as well.

Sleep hygiene

Sleep is a learned behavior. I recommend that you encourage babies to start learning about healthy sleep by putting them in their cribs, on their backs, full, dry, and drowsy but **awake**. Try not to allow the baby to fall asleep in your arms. If you rock a baby to sleep, then they expect that they will need you to rock them back to sleep when they wake up during the night. What we want to teach our baby is that he/she can eventually self-comfort and fall back to sleep on his/her own. Otherwise, your baby will cry for you to rock them every time they wake, and everyone (including babies) wake at various points during the night. We all just roll over and go back to sleep. Babies need to learn this skill.

Good sleep hygiene means that you go to bed and get up about the same time, daily. There should be a routine which precedes bedtime: bath, bottle, book, and bed ritual. In this way, the child will understand that bedtime follows bath, bottle and book time. Be sure your baby gets up about the same time every day and is put to bed around the same time each evening.

Babies love routine, and they function best when they understand the daily rhythm. If you interfere with their nap time, they will be fussy and have a difficult time at bedtime as well. Keeping a child up later doesn't mean that they will sleep in later, but in fact, often means they may wake earlier, and not fully rested.

Some babies get their days and nights confused. They want to sleep all day and play all night. I often see this when breastfeeding mothers return to work. Since the infant is now unable to nurse during the day, they decide to sleep more during the day, and nurse more at night. Although this is a difficult situation for a working mom, the infants thrive. To readjust their schedule, I encourage the parents to gradually reset their schedules by keeping them awake more during the daytime, and gradually spacing the night time feedings. Offering frequent bottle feedings during the day may help as well. Having a daycare provider who will offer stimulation to encourage the child to have more awake time during the day helps as well. I must confess, although exhausted, I enjoyed those 3 a.m. feedings as I missed my baby during my work day. What mother doesn't want to comfort her infant child? It's built into us. Don't get me wrong, I was still exhausted and worked hard to get my baby back to sleep at night.

Also, consider your sleep routine. If your schedule varies greatly, so will your child's. As children prefer routine, this is disruptive to infants. The more you regulate your own sleep/wake cycle, the better your child will do. Try to go to bed, and get up around the same time daily, even on weekends. Be aware of your caffeine consumption, as that may affect your sleep schedule.

Recognize your baby's signs that they feel sleepy. They may yawn or rub their eyes. They may close their eyes briefly, then open them quickly again. They may stop feeding and shut their eyes. They may start to cry, fuss, and whine. My daughter would always start playing with a strand of hair when she was sleepy. Each child will give you individual clues. Start watching for these. You will learn your child's body language.

Sleep environment

We all like to think about sleeping in a nice quiet dark room. That environment does aid adults in finding blissful sleep. Some parents demand pristine silence in the household while their baby naps or sleeps. This can be challenging when there are chores to do, laundry to be done, a dishwasher which needs to run, or planes flying outside. It seems that those who demand silence are setting themselves up for a situation in which any small noise can awaken their sleeping angel. Most bustling households with several children are almost never quiet. The baby learns to adapt and can sleep through dinner dishes and homework arguments. Children are very adaptive and will learn to live in the environment in which they are raised. I'm not suggesting you blare loud music at your newborn, but don't feel like you need to tip toe around if the baby drifts off. We must live our lives, and noise is a part of life. You may want to try to minimize the noise level around dinner time, as that is when babies get the fussiest. Soft music and dim lighting can help calm the evening chaos.

Comfort

As we speak about self-comforting behavior, babies often suck their fingers or thumbs. Sucking doesn't always mean hunger. Babies will often suck for comfort. If you feel comfortable using a pacifier, I have no issue with this. Pacifiers are very helpful for babies who have established their feeding routines and are less than a year old. They help to calm and comfort the child. They also may decrease the risk of Sudden Infant Death Syndrome (SIDS also known as crib death). Most infants will voluntarily give up the pacifier around six to nine months, but if it is continued beyond that point it may become more difficult to get rid of. After about nine months, it is no longer physical comfort, but it becomes psychological comfort. We've all seen older toddlers with pacifiers, who are trying to talk around a binky. Best to take it away by nine months to spare yourself the challenge of fighting the "binky war" later.

Babies also obtain comfort from swaddling, feeding, and being rocked or swayed. It's a great investment to get a baby swing. These can be used after two months, when the baby can easily support their own head. Although I don't recommend that babies sleep in swings, they can be very comforting. Babies should not sleep in swings or car seats, as it can impede their airway.

Of course, all infants seem to fall asleep in the car (never leave any infant or child unattended in a car). Not to worry. I'm just saying that at night, they need to stretch out and lie on their backs. Imagine sleeping in an airplane seat (coach) compared to the comfort of your own bed. You get the picture.

Sleeping through the night

Mothers of babies who awaken frequently during the night (like me) are green with envy of those mothers whose babies sleep through the night easily. It is not an easy burden to bear. Continuing to get up night after night with a crying infant when you would rather be snuggly cuddled into your warm bed is beyond difficult. There is hope, even for those of us with difficult sleepers. Sleeping through the night is defined by many texts as five to six hours of consecutive sleep. Most babies will "sleep through" by six months of age, if not before. Some babies will sleep through by three months. Although I wasn't that lucky, I hope you are. Before they reach sleeping through the night, babies still need to feed during the night.

There is a philosophy of sleep training called the Ferber method. This method encourages many of the sleep hygiene routines previously discussed such as bath, bottle, book, bed. It teaches the parent to place the baby full, dry, **awake**, but drowsy in bed on their back, and leave the room. The child cries. You return at intervals to comfort, but not pick up the baby. You check the baby first after three minutes, then after five minutes, and then 10 minutes, etc. until the child falls asleep. The next night you may start at five minutes. The night after that, you start at 10 minutes, etc. Eventually the baby learns to find sleep on their own, and they feel safe knowing that you are there to check on them. The age at which you begin this training is up to you as a parent. Although some advocate that this training may be started as young as three months of age, it makes more sense to me to wait until the six to nine-month age range to begin. Most infants still need to feed during the night until six to nine-months old. Ultimately, it's your choice when and how you decide to teach your child to sleep through the night. Remember that night wakening is a stage that babies go through. Like all stages, it eventually passes. You will again be able to sleep peacefully through the night someday soon. Now that we've discussed sleep…I recommend a nap!

Key points:

- Children eventually sleep through the night.
- Parents should try to sleep when the baby sleeps.
- Splitting the night shift gives both partners six solid hours of sleep.
- Most babies sleep through the night by six months of age.
- Young babies take a morning nap and an afternoon nap.
- The morning nap may disappear between 9 and 18 months of age.
- Sleeping on the back with a pacifier decreases the risk of crib death.
- Remove padding/choking hazards from the crib.
- Co-sleeping is not recommended due to risk of suffocation.
- Room sharing with a separate sleep surface for baby is encouraged.
- Put babies to bed full, dry, drowsy, but awake and on their back.
- Sleep training, like the Ferber method, may help train a baby to sleep.

Chapter 4: Why are they still crying?

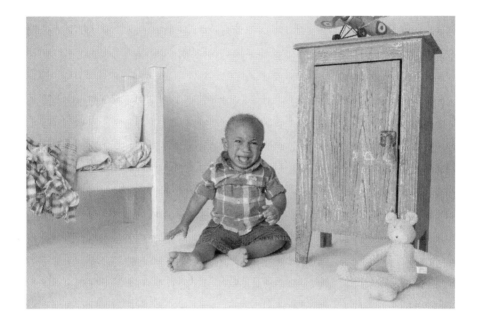

Raising Today's Baby

Chapter 4: Why are they still crying?

Congratulations! You're home with the baby. That's fantastic. Everyone's calling to wish you well. You're tired. You don't feel very well after the delivery…your breasts are swelling and the baby's crying and crying and crying. You've fed him/her, changed him/her and still there is crying, crying, crying. Well, after all crying is what babies do. It is natural. It is their one form of communication. Perhaps you haven't learned to speak baby yet? It's true that you WILL learn to distinguish between a hungry cry and a hurt cry. I didn't think I'd ever figure out what cry was what, but it comes to you after a bit.

Let us start with the basics.

Before I go into what you can do for your crying child, I want to share that I understand what you are going through. My first child, my son, was very colicky. He cried and cried, and then cried some more. The first few weeks were blurry with exhaustion and post-partum depression. When I finally came out of my "baby coma," there to welcome me was a crying infant. I felt so helpless and frustrated. After all, I had read all the books. I had a license as a registered nurse, and I had experience in pediatrics. Why wasn't my baby happy?

I tried everything. Sometimes I thought I might lose my mind. He was fussiest in the evening time when we were home from work. You can imagine that it was not the most pleasant time in our lives. I had pictured this wonderful life with a new baby. A baby who was constantly screaming was not exactly what I envisioned. After feeding, changing, and burping, still he cried and cried. I really understood the urge to shake a baby. But remember even a small amount of shaking can harm or even kill an infant. Thankfully, I had the self-control to lay him on his back in his crib and walk away. Many days that cup of tea downstairs was quite a comfort.

There is a suspended reality that occurs with pregnancy and childbirth. Preparing for pregnancy and birth is a magical time. It is a time of expectation, of hopes and dreams. You imagine your perfect baby and your perfect life. Then the birth happens, harder than you imagined, but manageable. You are then showered with company. Everyone gathers and celebrates joyfully. They give you gifts, cards, and flowers. It is wonderful. Then the celebration ends, and everyone goes home. So finally, here is the time you imagined. The beautiful, peaceful, loving time that you've anticipated with your new baby has arrived. Except that it is not beautiful OR peaceful, and you don't feel loving; you feel exhausted. It's hard being a new parent. The baby is demanding and cries and cries. You may feel helpless, hopeless, and fatigued. You are unable to do the one thing that you want to do most: soothe your own baby. You may feel defeated, like a failure. The mind-numbing exhaustion that sets in makes you feel depleted, both physically and emotionally. You need sleep, and you need it now. You need a break. But there is no break, no rest, no end in sight, so you push on. There are only feedings, changing, burping, rocking, cleaning and repeating every three hours. All you want is a happy healthy baby, but the baby wails. You can't seem to manage to fix things, so you feel inadequate, like you MUST be doing something wrong.

Reality sinks in. This is really it. This is what it means to be a parent. There must be a mistake. You've never seen this on a TV sitcom. While we all absolutely love our babies and are overjoyed to have them, the first few months can be so very difficult and challenging. No one really prepares you for these trying times, or helps you learn to manage the stress. These days can be really, really difficult. Not at all as wonderful as you had hoped and dreamed. Yet, there will be moments of redemption. Moments in the middle of the night, when the baby will coo or smile and suddenly you will realize that you are the only person in the world who just experienced joy from this angel. Please realize that it's not all bad. It is honestly the best and worst of times. Babies are wonderful. They change your life for the better, but sometimes they can be extremely challenging to live with. They can push you to places you've never been. They can bring you to joy that only a parent can know.

I really feel for single parents going through this. It can be exhausting to be the ONLY caregiver in this situation. Although married, I often got a taste of the lifestyle of a single parent, as my husband would deploy with the Navy, for up to six months at a time. I am thankful he was home to help for most of the child rearing, but during those deployments, I learned about going it alone. Back to that saying, "It takes a village to raise a child." This is the time to build your village of support. Neighbors, friends, co-workers, relatives all can be supportive of you and your child. Don't think that you must go it alone. Build that support by joining a parents' support group, a church parenting group or playgroup, and then make friends. These folks can help you immensely. You can trade child care services. Their emotional support may be all the help you need. I had arranged for childcare at a daycare when I headed back to work. Because my husband was gone, I also had two back-up plans in case of illness or other unknown disaster. A friend agreed to be my back-up person, and I was hers. In case she was unable to help, I had another friend waiting in the wings. It sounds silly, but if your child has a runny nose and you cannot miss another day of work, it helps. Sometimes you get stuck at work and need someone to pick-up your child at daycare for you. The result was that I survived the deployments and developed friendships that survive and prosper to this day. You can't buy that kind of relationship. These are people that I can trust and respect. You will need these folks to help you through the tough times and to rejoice in the joy a child brings. I would encourage you to develop relationships that are fulfilling and helpful. These types of relationships form bond stronger than that of blood. Families can be helpful as well. Don't hesitate to reach out to an aunt or cousin who would love a couple of hours of snuggle bug time.

If you think no one understands what you are experiencing, be assured you are not alone. Many parents, including myself, have been through this. Yes, I have slept on the floor next to the crib many a night. Talk to friends, neighbors, and relatives. I bet many of them can sympathize and help. The good news is that crying passes with time. My son's crying was helped with an infant swing. It also helped when I could accept that I couldn't stop all the crying. Crying doesn't harm a child. He survived, as did I, and so will you. Now read on to gain some insight on things you can do to manage, if not stop, your child's crying.

All babies cry. But how much, how long? The "experts" vary in their descriptions of "normal" crying. Most sources say that the average baby cries between one to four hours/day, but others disagree, arguing that even four to six hours a day is within the range of "normal." The average crying time for a two-week-old infant is 1 hour 45 minutes, while a six-week-old has an average crying time of 2 hours 45 minutes. Who really cares how long is normal when you are at your wits' end? Only parents know what it is really like to go through the frustration of a crying baby.

What we do know is that all babies cry. They cry to communicate. They cry when they are hungry, tired, want to be picked up, want to be put down, are wet, or sometimes just because they can. Crying can mean discomfort, over-stimulation, under-stimulation, too warm, too cool, illness, or teething.

The peak crying time is between 3 p.m. and 11 p.m. This busy evening time seems to affect babies the most. Crying does NOT hurt the baby. In fact, it is a normal, healthy response. Babies have many different cries which you will learn to interpret in time. You will find out that a painful cry sounds different from a hungry cry. Crying is your baby's first language. A cry is supposed to elicit a response from you…that's its job.

One of our many jobs as parents is to begin the process of teaching our child. The first lesson is that if the baby needs you, you will be there. This gives the child a sense of safety in the world, a sense of dependability. The baby thinks, if I'm uncomfortable, I cry and then these nice people (I'll call them angels, but they're also known as parents) come along and meet my needs (a bottle, a diaper change, a cuddle, a burp). The baby then grows up feeling safe and secure. The world is a very dependable place. The baby has some control over the world by being able to need assistance, ask for it, and receive it. This is the first and very important step to being able to build a normal emotional state. You cannot SPOIL a baby by tending to his/her cries.

But how can you tell WHY the baby is crying? It takes time and experience, something you may be short on right now. Let's again start with the basics. The baby is crying, and you don't know why. I would suggest taking a step approach to the crying:

Step 1: *Hungry?*

Could the baby be hungry? If it has been at least two and a half hours since the baby has eaten last, the baby may be hungry. New babies eat every two to three hours, older babies every three to four hours. Go ahead and try the breast/bottle, it often works. I do discourage feeding more often than every two hours in a newborn (or every three hours in a baby older than two months). I see many parents in the office who are feeding every hour or two because the child is crying. They don't realize that feeding too frequently may be contributing to the crying…ever eat too much at a holiday dinner? You may wonder if your baby is getting enough: watch for at least six wet diapers/day for infants over a week of age and have your baby weighed routinely as directed by your healthcare provider. Newborns usually consume one to two ounces of formula every two and a half to three hours, while older babies increase their feeds by age and weight.

If your child has fed, then why is he/she still crying? Some babies just need to suck for comfort, so try a pacifier. There are many different brands, and sometimes you need to try several brands to find one that a baby prefers.

Step 2: Wet?

Check the diaper. This is an easy fix, one not usually overlooked by new parents. Still in your fatigue, you might miss it. Dry pants never hurt! Is there a diaper rash? Irritated skin can be very uncomfortable. Try a diaper rash cream to soothe the rash. Avoid using diaper wipes which may burn irritated skin. Something as simple as a diaper change or some diaper cream may just solve the issue.

Step 3: Gassy?

Still crying? Perhaps you didn't get a good burp after that last feed. Often parents burp far too gingerly as if they were tapping a china doll. You need to cause enough stimulation to generate a decent burp, but never shake a baby. Gas in little tummies can cause crying. If you notice a lot of gas, try improving your burping techniques. Cup your hand and use your wrist to firmly pat the child's back for several minutes until he/she burps. NEVER

SHAKE a baby, but you must pat firmly. After a good burp, the baby may be able to rest.

Step 4: Colic?

Has the crying continued? We've fed, burped and changed this baby! You'd think we've met all his/her needs!!! Why is he/she still crying??? Well babies do tend to cry NORMALLY for several hours each day! Crying more than "average" is often called "colic." This term is poorly defined in the medical literature but relates to a fussy baby. We DO know that these fussy periods are more frequent in the evening hours and may be due to fatigue, over-stimulation, under-stimulation or frequent handling. If you've ever walked on crutches, you can imagine how sore little underarms can feel from constant handling. Sometimes a baby is just "over it" in the evening.

Baby-Wearing

There are many soothing activities for a baby with colic which we will discuss. Baby-wearing is one of them. Baby carriers allow parents to "wear" the baby, which leaves parents' hands free. The baby is comforted by the motion and warmth of Mom or Dad. The baby feels secure, like in the womb, and is calmed. Swaddling can also accomplish this. Babies do not like to feel loose. They want to be snuggled. If you choose to wear your baby, take precautions to position the head and neck in a safe position, and observe the infant closely. Be sure that the infant has good air supply. There are baby wearer support groups which meet regularly for dinner and a meeting. You may find a great support group by looking into this in your hometown.

Check out some resources online for baby wearing:
- BabywearingInternational.org
- TheBabywearer.com
- BabyCarrierIndustryAlliance.org
- BabywearingSchool.com

Step 5: Too Warm? Too Cold?

Check the temperature. Baby's rooms should be "room temperature" or a little cooler. Do not over-dress the child. The child should be dressed just like you are. If you are in shorts and a tank, then just a t-shirt and diaper is fine. If you are in jeans and a sweater, then a long sleeve sleeper will do. Don't over-blanket the child. He/she may just be too warm. Feel the hands and feet. A cold child will have cold hands, as the hands give up the heat to warm the core. It may sound silly, but the baby may just be expressing that he/she is uncomfortable due to the temperature. An infant in a car can be too cold or too warm depending on the season. Always try to warm the car in the winter or cool the car in the summer prior to placing a baby in the car. It should go without saying, but never leave a child unattended in a car (not even for a few minutes), as they can overheat rapidly, and may die. This can happen in a matter of minutes. No errand is worth your child's life. Sadly, I hear of this very situation on the news every summer. Temperature concerns may cause crying, as your baby is saying "I'm too warm or too cold…please help me."

Step 6: Over-Stimulated?

Some babies are over-stimulated. These babies do not like loud noises or bright lights. They are sensitive to the activity around them. They calm during dim lighting and quiet. Sometimes, they just want to be left alone in the crib. Instead of a busy dinnertime with the TV blaring, try a quiet evening atmosphere, darkened room and warm bath (never leave baby unattended in bath water). Give the baby a gentle massage (who wouldn't love that?) and leave him/her to lie alone in their crib on the back with the side rails up for 15 to 20-minute intervals, checking frequently on him/her. Try giving the pacifier as well. Remember the AAP recommends the back-sleeping position (with pacifier use) to decrease the risk of Sudden Infant Death Syndrome (SIDS). Leave the room and shut the door. Take a break...have a cup of tea, watch some TV, go downstairs. After a few minutes quietly peek in to check the baby...you may be surprised! If he/she continues crying after 20 to 30 minutes, go back to step one and recheck steps one to four.

Step 7: Under-Stimulated?

Other babies are under-stimulated. They love noise and activity. They soothe to music and motion. Consider taking a car ride. First, safely strap the baby into an approved car seat (backwards facing until age two) in the back seat. Try using an infant swing or try walking and rocking the baby. I do not advocate getting into the habit of rocking the baby to sleep every time, unless you don't mind rocking all night...since whenever the baby awakens, he/she will demand to be rocked back to sleep. Who wants to be driving around all night in a car, just to soothe the baby? Try a mobile over the crib or some musical toy. Some of the cribs now have a vibrating component which some infants adore.

Step 8: Disrupted Sleep/Eat Cycle?

Have you been traveling? Did the baby get on a different schedule after visiting Grandma? I see many babies in the office who get off schedule following a trip or a visit. Sometimes, even brief visits can upset a baby's sleeping and eating schedule. To get them back to normal, try to keep your baby on a regular sleeping and eating cycle. I recommend feedings every three hours during the day (6, 9, 12, 3, 6). Try to limit morning naps to one to two hours, and afternoon naps to no more than two to three hours, so this can regulate the day/night cycle. Newborns will need to eat every three hours around the clock, and sometimes more frequently. If the baby's schedule is way off course, adjust the feeding times by 15 to 30 minutes each day until you are back on track. Babies really want a regular routine. This helps them to predict and anticipate their day. I don't know if you've ever been somewhere where you don't have control of your schedule: you are not sure what's going to happen next. As an exchange student in Switzerland, I didn't speak the language and often felt like I wasn't sure what the plan for the day might be. It's an unsettling feeling. You are at the mercy of someone else, much like an infant is at the mercy of the parent's care. Giving them a sense of schedule and predictability may help.

Step 9: Ill?

For a baby that doesn't respond to comforting, seek medical care. Seek immediate medical care for an infant with a temperature at or above 100.4 degrees (especially prior to two months of age). Is the child ill? Could there be a fever? Is the cry piercing? Does it sound like the baby is in pain? If the crying seems excessive or persistent, call your healthcare provider immediately for evaluation. Note if there is a certain time of day or position that increases the crying. Is there arching? Pulling up of the legs? Pulling of the ears? Keep a log of the times and issues that your child is having. This will help your healthcare provider make an accurate diagnosis. Your healthcare provider will then provide you with a diagnosis and options for treatment if necessary. Babies can have infections which cause illness, such as a urinary tract infection, ear infection, or even more serious infections. They could have experienced trauma, perhaps falling or having been shaken. Sometimes, parents are not aware of such incidents if the baby has been cared for by someone else. There can be gastrointestinal issues, such as reflux, or constipation. There can be nutritional issues, such as overfeeding, underfeeding, or milk/soy protein allergies. There can be skin issues, such as eczema, diaper rash, insect bites, tight clothing, or hair encircling a finger or toe. They can be teething, or just have simple colic. Babies can cry for many reasons. If you are not sure why your baby is crying, a medical examination is strongly recommended.

Seek help

If things are difficult for you right now, find a healthcare provider that you trust and someone who will listen to you. You want to develop a relationship with a healthcare provider which will last 20 years. If you feel you are not being heard, seek care elsewhere. Ask your friends, family, and neighbors. Word of mouth is the very best referral. If you feel you are being brushed off, try another provider within the group. Some folks just "gel" better with one provider over another. You want someone who will listen to your concerns and address them. I try to teach my students that if they want to know what's wrong with the baby, ask the parent. Parents know their children better than anyone else in the world. If you listen long enough to the parent, then you will find out what the problem is. Sometimes communication between the provider and the parent is the most important aspect of the medical visit.

Reaching your limit

Everyone reaches a limit. This limit happens when you have done everything you know to do, and the baby still cries. I understand. I've been there. It's important to know what to do when you reach this limit. It usually occurs when you are tired and frustrated. No matter how frustrated you become, please remember: **NEVER SHAKE A BABY!!!!!** Even short shaking can cause shaken baby syndrome which causes blindness, severe brain damage and…even death. It is NEVER okay to shake a baby. If you can't deal with the crying any longer then it's time to gently lie the baby in his/her crib on his/her back (put the pacifier in his/her mouth) with the side rails up and leave the room. Call a friend, relative or neighbor. Ask for some help…even a few minutes break to "run to the store" may help to reset your mind. Of course, never leave a child unattended, but you don't have to be in the same room every second of the day. It is okay to give yourself permission for a 10 or 15-minute break. Remember this stage isn't forever. Colic is a stage which generally improves in a few months (usually by 12 weeks of life). These children are normal, healthy, well-adjusted children. I can remember laying my son in his crib, shutting the door, and going downstairs to sit on the front step for just a moment of peace. After composing myself, I could attend to his needs once again. Thankfully, although he was an inconsolable baby, he was a very easy child to raise as he got older and is now a delightful young man.

Crying is normal

Crying is a normal part of raising a child. It communicates their needs. It lets them know that the world is a dependable place where their needs will be met. It lets them know that they are safe. Remember that it doesn't hurt a baby to cry. It is, in fact, good for them to cry sometimes. It increases their oxygenation, exercises their lungs, increases their heart rates, and communicates their needs. Essentially, crying is the only way babies can communicate those needs. They need to know that we as parents understand their needs and will meet those needs. Once we have done everything we know how to do, we take a break and then try again. Remember: THIS TOO SHALL PASS!

Here are some suggestions to soothe a fussy baby:

- Rocking
- Gently sway
- Swaddling

- A car ride (backwards facing, in an infant car seat)
- Swinging
- White noise (fan/vacuum)
- Pacifier
- Warm bath
- Gentle massage
- Darkened or dim room
- Quiet
- Soft gentle music
- Carrying (in a baby carrier)
- Walking with baby
- Going outside
- Stroller ride

Still crying?

Finally, calm yourself. Babies can sense your emotions. If you are stressed and frazzled, they will feel this. A happy baby needs a happy, relaxed, controlled, and focused parent/caregiver. Take a break. Get a sitter and go out to dinner. Get a massage. Ask for some help and then accept the help.

You are not the only person who can do dishes, cooking, cleaning, and laundry. Get some exercise. Talk to friends. You can survive this difficult time. Try to remember this fussy phase as a brief stage which is mostly joyful. I promise that when this child is five years old, we will be talking about different problems.

Depressed?

So, if you are in a dark place: if you feel hopeless, helpless, and alone, please seek help. Start by admitting these feelings to yourself (and your family) and then get help, both professional and personal. Postpartum depression is a real thing and can be managed with therapy and sometimes medication. Start by speaking with your OB/GYN healthcare provider or a mental health specialist. There should be a 1-800 number on the back of your insurance card for mental health services. If you need to speak to someone immediately, call the **National Suicide Prevention Lifeline at 1-800-273-8255**. Also, seek help through family and friends. Remember your family and friends love you and care about you. They want only the best for you and your child. They would love to be helpful to you. You may be surprised at how willing they are to assist you. Even having them take the baby out for a carriage ride may give you a chance to have an hour nap.

Sometimes a nap can do wonders. But seriously, see a mental health professional if you are depressed. Your child needs you.

Self-care

Above all, don't forget to take care of yourself. Too often, we focus on caring for our children but neglect our own needs. We cannot be optimal parents if our needs are not met. Try to split feedings so that both partners can get six hours of uninterrupted sleep (mom sleeps from 9 p.m. to 3 a.m. and dad sleeps from 12 a.m. to 6 a.m.). Eat as healthily as possible. Remember fruits and vegetables? Take your vitamins. Drink lots of water. Take a walk. I can remember just wishing for time to take a shower. You need to take care of yourself as well as your baby. Review Chapter 2 on finding balance as a parent.

Feed your soul

Find something you love to do that feeds your soul and do it. Read a book, paint a picture, write a poem, call a friend, walk on the beach, hike in the hills, plant some flowers, sing a song, or do a dance. Even a single flower may bring you joy. Rediscover your inner joys. You will want to pass these joys to your children. Keep them alive. Include some time for stress relief. Take a warm bath. Get a massage. Steep the perfect cup of tea. Cozy up in a soft blanket. Light a fragrant candle. Have someone give you a foot massage (my personal favorite). You are the only one who can really care for you, so do it. Your child needs you to be healthy, happy and whole for you to be the best parent possible. Caring for yourself strengthens you and allows you to adequately care for your child. Above all, realize that this short season of crying is only a brief time in your life. Brighter days are ahead…I promise.

Key points:

- Babies normally cry about one to four hours each day.
- Crying is a baby's only means of communication.
- Crying does not harm a baby.
- Babies have different cries for different needs.
- You cannot spoil a baby by responding to their crying.
- Never shake a baby.
- If frustrated, lay the baby on their back in the crib with the side rails up and leave the room.
- Babies cry when they are hungry, wet or gassy.
- Babies cry when they are too warm or too cold.
- Babies cry when they are over or under-stimulated.
- Babies cry when their sleep/eating cycle is disrupted.
- Babies cry when they are ill.
- Colic is crying more than normal and passes around 12 weeks of age.
- Rocking, carrying, baths, swings, and car rides may calm your baby.
- Address any concerns of depression with a mental health professional.
- Care for yourself so that you will be able to care for your child.

Raising Today's Baby

Chapter 5: Bath time and bubbles

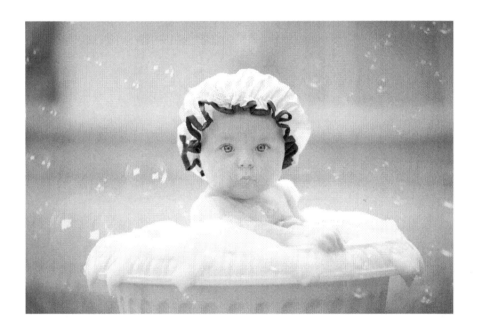

Raising Today's Baby

Chapter 5: Bath time and bubbles

I adored bath time with my children. Particularly when they were babies, as they loved to splash and play. Allow me a moment to paint a scene. It's the evening of an ordinary day. Dinner is finished, and the kitchen is clean (okay, now I'm really dreaming). We pick up the night's toys and head to the bathroom. The baby is playful, even laughing out loud as she splashes with the bath toys. There are rubber ducks, boats, and at times even a naked Barbie; after all, Barbie needs to bathe as well. The baby shampoo bubbles as I form a peak-like mountain with the sparse hair on my sweet daughter's head. I get a two-toothed grin and am accidentally splashed in the face. I chuckle. I can hear the TV downstairs, and the sound of my family settling in for the evening. My son runs down the hall. Still, for a moment, it's peaceful, just me and the baby for bath time. We sing and splash. I brush her little teeth. I wash her tiny face; I notice her grimace and appreciate her tolerance. She does not enjoy the rinsing of her hair, but the moment passes, and life catches up with me. Time to get out of the tub. Time for jammies, book, and bed. Her face is so clean that her cheeks are rosy. Her hair squeaks as I dry it.

After their baths, my babies smelled like angels: fresh and wonderful. Even their breath was sweet. I'd comb their hair into small peaks on the tops of their heads to make curls with a soft brush, which seemed doll-sized. I applied lotion. I put a footie sleeper on the baby.

Why does it feel so good to snuggle babies after bath time? You just want to hold and rock them. It makes us, as parents, feel wonderful. That evening bottle (or breastfeeding) is a delight as you breathe in their clean scent and look at their wet hair. You almost can't put them down after the bottle is gone. This is one of the rewards of parenting, and despite all the challenges and difficulties, this is what makes it all worthwhile. For a few minutes you get to spend time with the most precious child in the world…yours. For one brief moment, in a quiet bath, you get to hear the sound of laughter which is just for you. You are the recipient of that private laugh and smile. You share the intimate moments before bedtime. Please, do yourself a favor and make the most of these precious moments. They pass far too quickly.

I had so many questions about bathing and skin care. I wondered what soap to use, and whether to use lotion. Why did it matter what detergent I used? How hot should the water be? How often do babies need a bath?

When can I bathe my newborn?

Babies need to be bathed. Skin care is a great concern for new parents. First, new parents wonder when they can bathe their new baby. Generally, a tub or even a sink bath is not recommended until after the umbilical cord falls off. The umbilical cord needs to dry to fall off, and this cannot happen if we are dipping the baby into water. The cord usually comes off between two and three weeks of age. Meanwhile, it is okay to wash the baby gently with a dye-free, fragrance-free non-soap cleanser (Dove unscented, Cetaphil or Johnson-Johnson unscented are among my favorites).

How do I clean the umbilical cord?

Years ago, the recommendation was to cleanse the umbilical cord twice daily with water or rubbing alcohol. The current recommendation is to do nothing to the cord. Honestly, doing nothing seems to work fine. I used rubbing alcohol with both my children, but that was the medical recommendation at that time. You may want to discuss this issue with your pediatric healthcare provider, as recommendations change from time to time. Doing nothing is the current recommended course of action. Just keep the cord dry (no tub baths until the cord falls off). The cord usually comes off within two weeks.

Never leave a child unattended in the tub

Be sure to NEVER leave any child unattended (alone) in the tub or near any water! Babies, especially toddlers can drown in less than an inch of water in just a few minutes. Babies are "head heavy", in other words their heads are heavier than other parts of their bodies. If they fall into a tub, a toilet, a washing machine or a bucket with a small amount of water in it, they are unable to get back out. They get stuck "head down" and may drown trying to get out. NEVER leave any child unattended around any water. Even an inch of water in a container can be deadly in just a moment.

Safety must be the priority in bathing. Be aware that wet, soapy babies are slippery. Use an infant tub chair for added ease and safety. Be sure to have all the necessary materials on hand before you begin. You will need shampoo, soap, a wash cloth, two towels, the tub chair, lotion, diaper, diaper cream, and PJs. If you are alone and giving the baby a bath, wear sensible shoes. Socks can get slippery when wet. Bring the phone with you into the bathroom. There should be no reason to have to leave the bathroom, so if the phone is with you, you won't be tempted to leave. Otherwise, just ignore the ring. No phone call is worth your baby's life, as babies can drown quickly. Also, the phone is nice to have in case of any emergency. Remember, even if your child sits well, do NOT leave him/her unattended in the water. Babies can lose their balance, tumble over, and drown quickly. Babies can tumble and bump their heads. Safety is an important issue in the bath. Bath toys such as ducks or boats make bath time fun and educational. Babies can learn about how things float and move in the water.

Bathing tips

If you have a newborn, I suggest you get a tub chair which the baby reclines on during the bath. Babies can also be bathed in the sink. Older infants who can sit up do well sitting in a laundry basket placed in the tub for support. (Again, NEVER leave them unattended!) Always check the water temperature prior to placing the infant in the water! For safety reasons, your water heater should be set no higher than 120 degrees F to prevent scalding injuries. Unfortunately, some parents may run the bath water without checking it and place the baby in water that is too hot. These babies can be burned severely by water that is too hot. Remember babies can't tell you if the water is too warm or too cool. They depend on you to determine the appropriate water temperature. You will want the water to be warm to the touch but not burning. Place your hand submerged to your wrist for a few moments to check the water temperature. It should feel warm and comfortable to the touch, not hot. You'll need just enough lukewarm water to cover the baby up to his/her stomach. Be careful and remember: wet babies are slippery and soapy babies even more so!

What should I use to wash the baby?

Wash the baby gently using a dye-free, fragrance-free cleanser, such as Dove unscented or Cetaphil cleanser. Aveeno also has a nice cleanser. I do not recommend antibacterial soap, which may be too irritating for sensitive baby skin. Also, antibacterial soaps contain triclosan, which can increase bacterial resistance. There is discussion that antibacterial products containing triclosan should be banned. Start with the top and work down. Be sure your shampoo is gentle, such as Johnson and Johnson head-to-toe. Wash an area, then rinse the area. Dry that area, then move on. After bathing, use a dye-free, fragrance-free lotion such as Cetaphil, Eucerin, Lubriderm, or Aveeno. Avoid products that contain lavender or tea tree oil, which may irritate sensitive skin. There is also some thought that tea tree oil can cause unwanted hormonal changes. Best to avoid these in children.

What about organic products?

There are many products on the market that are directed for babies. Some of the terms can be confusing or misleading. The term natural is not the same as organic. The term organic is regulated by the National Organic Standards Board, according to the Organic Food Production Act of 1990. "Made with only organic ingredients" means that 70% of the materials are certified as organic. The USDA Organic Seal mean that at least 95% of the ingredients are organic. You can review the USDA website for organic labeling yourself.

Although I love the concept of natural and organic products, I sometimes find them to be somewhat misleading. I think an all-natural world would be lovely, however, am I buying what I think I am buying, or are they misleading me with advertising? I usually recommend baby products which are dye-free, and fragrance-free. Just because something is organic doesn't mean it won't irritate sensitive baby skin. Organic products can be made from natural products which may have fragrance, such as lavender. These fragrances may irritate sensitive skin. I recommend products which are not expensive and therefore easily affordable for most patients. My favorite baby soap is Dove unscented. My favorite lotions include Cetaphil,

Lubriderm, Aveeno, or Eucerin. I recommend emollients such as Vaseline (unscented) or Aquaphor to be placed on top of the lotion for dry areas. The emollient traps the moisture in. I use Vitamin A+D, Desitin, or Butt Paste as diaper creams. It's fine if you choose to use a natural or organic product but understand that you may be paying for the label. The choice in infant products is entirely up to you. You can see how your baby's skin responds to different products. If you have an issue, please consult your healthcare professional.

Other organic labels which you may encounter:

DEMETER: This global non-profit group requires that 90% of ingredients come from farms that are organic and sustainable.

ECOCERT: This independent European based group uses the labels of organic cosmetic and natural cosmetic. Both require 95% of ingredients come from natural origins. The organic cosmetic also requires that 10% of ingredients come from organic farming, while natural cosmetic requires only 5%.

LEAPING BUNNY: This animal rights group seal means that no new animal testing is used during product development.

NPA: Natural Products Association for beauty and home care products are composed of 95% "natural" ingredients. By natural they mean coming from a renewable source in nature.

NSF/ANSI 305: The National Sanitation Foundation and the American National Standards Institute monitors many things including that the product is at least 70% organic.

What's that in the tub?

Don't be surprised if your child pees or poops in the water. Try not to freak. It is very natural. All children do this at one time or another. (Yes, I'll agree that it is gross.) Remember, they do not have control over their bladder or bowels yet, so there is no sense yelling or scolding a baby for this. If they peed, just continue the bath, as urine is sterile. It will not hurt them. If they pooped, you will want to rinse them off, lift them out of the water, wrap them in a towel, and declare bath time over. After drying, applying lotion, and clothing, the baby can be placed safely in the crib with the side rails up.

You can then go back and clean up the tub. Let the water drain. Use a zip lock baggie or a plastic grocery bag as a glove to lift the poo from the tub and place it (the poo, not the plastic bag) into the toilet. Dispose of the plastic bag in the trash. Spray the tub with bleach to kill any bacteria. Rinse well. Life goes on. Poop happens. Fact of life, babies poop in the tub. Try not to stress. If this topic completely freaks you out, try not to bathe your baby right after feeding, as you may be more likely to get poo after meal time.

Circumcision care

If you choose to have circumcision for your son, you can use Vaseline or Vaseline plus Neosporin to aid healing and prevent the raw area from sticking to the diaper. There is no such thing as too much Vaseline around this raw area. Expect a yellow-white moist scab after discharge from the hospital. There is no need to clean this area, just let it heal. Be sure to point the penis downward in the diaper to prevent diaper leakage around the belly. After the area heals on your circumcised son, be sure to gently pull back the foreskin to cleanse around the glans or head of the penis. You don't want to force this. Be gentle. In uncircumcised boys, the foreskin may not retract completely, but it will stretch in time. Your pediatrician will evaluate this.

It normally will retract fully by the time the boy enters puberty, but if there are concerns an elective circumcision may be scheduled. Also, remember when cleaning your son to gently lift the testicles, as there can be stool products lodged beneath the testicles, which can irritate sensitive skin.

Whether or not to have your son circumcised is a personal decision, one that is best made by yourself and your family. It's not a required procedure, and certainly many folks opt out. For some, circumcision is part of their faith. There are also some medical reasons to circumcise. It can lead to easier hygiene, and therefore less infection in the foreskin area. It can help prevent phimosis which is a narrowing of the foreskin. It may slightly decrease your son's risk of urinary tract infections. It also may decrease the risk of sexually transmitted diseases and HIV/AIDS. There are some reasons not to circumcise. It is painful. It is a procedure which opens the skin so there is a slight risk of infection. Newer medical data leans toward the benefits of circumcision but ultimately, the choice is yours.

Female hygiene

On girls, cleanse the vaginal folds but avoid the inner vaginal area, which can be very sensitive. Be sure to open the labial area and inspect, so that you are familiar with the normal appearance of the baby's genitalia. That way, you can watch for any problems. Sometimes the girls have "labial adhesions," or labia that are partly fused together. This will usually resolve without intervention by the age of three years. If the area is completely closed, your pediatrician may recommend a hormone cream (Premarin) to open the area. It is not necessary to dig into your daughter's vaginal area to clean, just a gentle wipe over the area should suffice.

Cradle cap

Sometimes babies will get a crusty scalp. This is called cradle cap. If your baby is having any problems with cradle cap, which would appear as a flaky yellow crust on the top of the head, this likely will resolve in time as the scalp matures. Often, nothing needs to be done for this. If you wish, you can use over-the-counter Selsun Blue Shampoo twice a week until it clears. Lather it on the scalp being careful to avoid the eyes. Allow it to set for a few minutes while you finish the bath, then rinse off. Afterward, apply a bit of unscented baby oil to moisturize the scalp and use a soft baby brush to massage or remove the flakes. Pat the scalp dry and place the baby oil on within 30 seconds to prevent the scalp from drying any further. It may take several weeks to get this condition under control.

Sensitive skin

After bathing, dry the infant well with a towel and apply a dye-free, fragrance-free moisturizer such as Eucerin, Lubriderm, or Cetaphil due to baby's sensitive skin. If the baby has any dry bumpy or peeling areas, I'd also use an emollient over the lotion such as Vaseline (fragrance-free of course) or Aquaphor. Vaseline may be used up to four times/day. "Soaking and greasing" is an effective way to control dry skin. Again, patting the skin dry and applying the lotion quickly, within minutes, is the most effective way to keep the moisture in and prevent over-drying of the skin.

I have very sensitive skin, as do most babies. Sensitive skin rashes easily and becomes irritated with products that contain fragrances or dyes. Be sure to also use a dye-free, fragrance-free detergent on ALL your families' clothes (not just the baby's) such as "Cheer free" or "All free and clear."

Remember, your baby's face is on your shirt most of the time! It's important that your clothing be non-irritating to the baby's sensitive skin. Also, be aware that perfumes or scented lotions that you are wearing may irritate the baby. Babies love to snuggle in the folds of our neck, where we usually spray our perfume. Be aware of any cosmetics or lotions on your hands, as babies love to suck fingers. Be sure to wash your hands thoroughly with soap and water before handling infants. Most germs are carried and passed via our hands, so cleanliness of the hands is crucial to good health.

Diaper wipes

Diaper wipes are handy and convenient but may be irritating to baby's sensitive skin. They are not meant to be used to wipe tiny faces and hands, but I see them used often as wash cloths. I do not recommend this as it may irritate the infant's face. Just a warm clean wash cloth does a great job on faces. I only use diaper wipes if the child stools. We don't wash each time we urinate, and the child doesn't really need to be wiped that often either. Too frequent wiping with diaper wipes can irritate a little bottom. If the baby is just wet, just change the diaper. If they have stooled, then use the wipe. If they have a bad diaper rash, forgo the wipe and use just water and a clean wash cloth, as the diaper wipe may further irritate a diaper rash. Use the wipes sparingly. It's easy to place a wet washcloth in a plastic bag in the diaper bag for quick touch-ups while on the go.

Diaper cream

There are many diaper creams on the market. As I've said, Vitamin A+D ointment and Butt Paste are among my favorites. I like the Vitamin A+D as it is transparent (clear) and you can monitor any rash easily. There is also a clear Desitin, but it does not contain zinc oxide. If you have a rash with a raw area, Desitin or Butt paste which contain zinc oxide sticks particularly well. Any product with zinc oxide will work. Apply cream at every diaper change if there is a rash.

Eczema

If you have a family history of eczema (also called atopic dermatitis), it is especially important for baby to avoid fragrances and dyes. Also remember that eczema has been shown to be linked to allergies and asthma. Eczema is dry, itchy skin. It often appears as small red bumps on cheeks, ankles, behind the knees, folds of the arms, and behind the neck. It can appear as discolored patches on the tummy or back. It is rough to the touch. It can be managed by using dye-free, fragrance-free soaps, lotions, and emollients (such as Vaseline). Additional prescription medication, such as topical steroid creams are sometimes necessary. If you are concerned about a rash or dry irritated skin on your child, always consult your healthcare professional.

Bathing frequency

Parents ask me how often they should bathe their babies. Bathing can be done daily or every other day. I always bathed my children daily once the umbilical cord had fallen off, but I know many folks who bathe their children every second or third day. Other countries do not bathe themselves or their children nearly as often as Americans do. It is perfectly acceptable to bathe your infant every other, or even every third day. I would not recommend bathing less than twice per week, as their sensitive skin can become irritated. Some folks worry about bathing their infant if he/she is ill. A bath is fine, but we don't want the child to become chilled. Also, if they have a fever, a warm bath can cool and comfort the child, however, it is important to use a warm bath to prevent a too rapid change in temperature. Again, not allowing the child to be chilled is key.

The length of the bath is important, as babies can lose heat quickly. Babies do not regulate their temperature as well as adults. Therefore, babies wear hats. The hats help them avoid heat loss from the head. Especially young babies need to be kept warm, but not over-heated. They can very easily get chilled during bath time. Be sure to use an enclosed space to help avoid drafts. Be sure to use warm, comfortable water. Bathe quickly, rinse, and dry gently by patting to protect sensitive skin. Use two towels, one to cover the baby, and the other to dry areas. This helps to minimize heat loss. Lotion and dry the baby on a safe surface, as falls are one of the biggest health risks to an infant. Quickly apply lotion to trap in moisture.

Rash?

Infant skin can often get bumps or a rash. Using dye-free, fragrance-free soaps, lotions, and detergents can help minimize this issue. If your child has a rash, see your pediatric healthcare provider for assistance. Often, a dye-free, fragrance-free lotion plus an emollient, such as Vaseline or Aquaphor, may be all that is needed. It's easy to become neurotic about every little bump, so try not to worry, but get things checked. Any rash with fever should be evaluated immediately by your healthcare provider.

Mani/pedi?

Nail trimming is always a concern. Babies' little nails can be sharp. They can scratch themselves easily. File or peel your child's nails. Newborns fingernails are very soft and will peel right off. As one (horrible) mother (I mean me), who accidentally clipped her newborn daughter's fingertip, making her bleed, I recommend a safer way…peel or file. A nail file works just as well and has less chance of bloodshed (the voice of experience). With older babies, sometimes it's easier to attempt nail care when they are asleep. Some recommend using baby mittens or socks over the hands to prevent scratching, but I prefer to allow those hands to be free. Those hands need to move and explore.

Comfort in the tub

Babies have different comfort levels with bathing and skin care. Some love water and splash, laugh, and play. Others may be afraid of it. I remember a child I cared for in the hospital, who had been burned severely in hot water.

I could not get that child into the tub. Finally, I rolled up my sleeves and I splashed in the water, laughing. Soon, the child crawled over and wanted in to play. Once she found out that the water wasn't scalding, she was all for it. Please be sure to check the water temperature before placing your child in any water, and never leave a child unattended in water, not even for a second.

Sensory issues

Children with sensory issues may become especially unhappy if placed in the water. If you find that you are having issues related to bath time that are unexpected or unusual, consult your pediatric healthcare provider. Look for signs such as fear of the water or bath, screaming with each bath (not just when they get their faces washed), or refusal to play during bath time. Talk about it with your healthcare provider. If you get brushed off, find a provider who will take the time to listen to you. You have valid concerns about your child that need to be heard. You know your child better than anyone else in the world. You will come to know your child's individual temperament about bath time. Even unhappy babies need to be bathed regularly. Talk to a professional if you have concerns. Ask them for age appropriate developmental screenings (these should be done regularly at your well examinations). Try to make bath time a relaxing and enjoyable experience for you and your child by planning ahead with supplies: toys, songs or music, and a playful attitude (warning: your clothes may get wet).

As we bathe our children, we get a wonderful rewarding sensation that we are taking care of their basic needs as well as making them feel good and relaxed, just as we do after a great shower. We are doing a good job as parents. We feel the same when we prepare a great healthy meal for our families, and we know we've given our child what they need to flourish and grow. Bath time is an intimate bonding time, which can be used for teaching songs, dental care, and hygiene habits. It's a special time of day to be enjoyed and cherished. Here's to happy and safe splashing!

Key points:

- Wait until the umbilical cord is off to give a tub bath.
- Never leave a child unattended in the tub.
- Water heaters should be set at 120 degrees F.
- Dye-free fragrance-free soaps, lotions, & detergents are best.
- Use diaper wipes sparingly and not on little faces.
- Vaseline works well for circumcision care.
- Avoid antibacterial soaps.
- Avoid products containing lavender or tea tree oil.
- File little nails to prevent over trimming.
- Safety first while bathing: keep supplies close.
- Always have the phone with you while bathing your infant in case of an emergency.

Raising Today's Baby

Chapter 6: Medical care 411

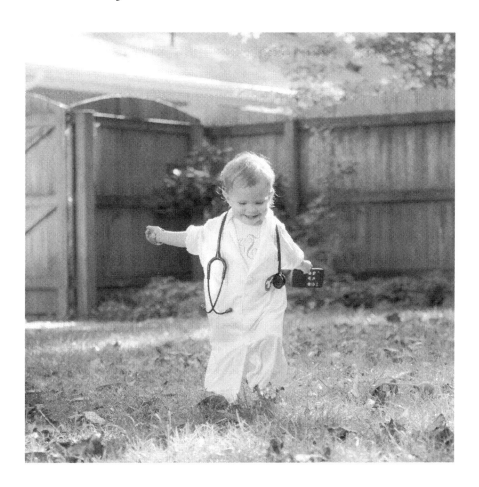

Raising Today's Baby

Chapter 6: Medical care 411

A very pregnant first-time mom once asked me how often she would be at the pediatric office during the first year. I told her it would seem like she was personal friends with ALL of us by the end of that year. Well visits are scheduled within 48 to 72 hours from hospital discharge at three to five days of life, between 2 and 4 weeks, and then 2, 4, 6, 9, 12, 15, 18, 24, 30, 36 months just for well visits. After that, well visits will be yearly. This doesn't even take account the visits when your child is ill. Maybe that's why I feel so close to so many families that I see.

Many parents wonder if the well visits are necessary. I would argue that not only are they necessary, but that they are urgently important. It is at these routine screenings that we most often catch and diagnose problems.

I've been asked if it's okay to go to a family medical practitioner or a family nurse practitioner. Although, family medical practitioners and family nurse practitioners are wonderful for adults, please understand that pediatric practices are devoted exclusively to children. Children are not small adults. They have different problems; they have different health issues, require different medications, and therefore need different healthcare providers. I strongly feel it is in your child's best interest to see a provider who is a specialist in pediatrics. Pediatric healthcare providers devote their life study only to children. Just as you would not go to an eye doctor for a heart issue, or a kidney doctor for a stomach issue, you should see the right specialist for your child. Not only have we studied ONLY pediatrics, but we must stay up to date with continuing education. Pediatrics changes rapidly. The advice we offer must change with the current research. No one person can stay up to date on all things, so you want someone who specializes in pediatrics. You want someone who is board certified in pediatrics. Experience is helpful as well. I recommend the very best in pediatric care for your most precious child by recommending a pediatric healthcare provider. There are pediatricians (MDs: medical doctors) and pediatric nurse practitioners (such as myself).

It is recommended to have a "medical home" for your child. This is their "regular" pediatric office. This allows one practice to keep up with your child's immunization status, growth records and past medical history. The medical home provides the best care for children by keeping track of specialist visits, lab results and records. You can then develop a relationship with that group of providers (or maybe find that one special provider). I encourage my patients to use their medical home for routine healthcare needs in lieu of urgent care centers where they may not know or understand your child's history. Of course, for emergent or after-hours situations, emergency departments or urgent care centers are available as well.

What is a Pediatric Nurse Practitioner?

I am often asked what a Pediatric Nurse Practitioner is. A nurse practitioner is a Registered Nurse with a bachelor's degree in nursing, who went back to school to get a master's degree in nursing. The DNP or Doctor of Nursing Practice is a relatively new degree for clinical nurse practitioners. There has been discussion that soon all new NPs will have to have their doctorate, either a DNP or a PhD. (Clinicians generally choose the DNP, while academics or researchers choose the PhD. Previous NPs will be grandfathered in, so they will not have to have a doctoral degree.) Also, you want to look for a Certified Pediatric Nurse Practitioner (CPNP) which means that they are board-certified in pediatrics and may practice as a CPNP.

Pediatric Nurse Practitioners (PNPs) perform both well exams as well as sick exams. PNPs function much like your pediatrician. PNPs can prescribe medication and provide excellent medical care for your child. Studies show that most people are as satisfied or more satisfied with a PNP as they are with a medical doctor (MD). Patient and parent education are particular strengths of the PNP. Often a PNP may see fewer patients per day, having more time to spend with each patient. The choice in healthcare providers is yours. Find a healthcare provider that is well educated, has experience, is board certified, and listens to your concerns. A Pediatric Nurse Practitioner may just fit that spot.

Prenatal care for expectant mothers

If you are currently expecting please allow me to remind you that your prenatal well examinations are essential to providing good prenatal care to your unborn child. It is vital that you care for yourself during these critical days of development and follow your obstetric healthcare provider's advice to the letter. Take your prenatal vitamins and keep up with your check-ups. Write your list of questions and take them with you. Ask about dietary and vitamin recommendations (including what you should avoid). I will leave this advice to your OB/GYN as they are the experts in this arena.

The well visit

There are two types of pediatric appointments: well visits and sick visits. The well visit is a much more detailed visit, whereas the sick visit focuses on the illness at hand. I recommend you come prepared to the baby's well visit. The baby will be weighed, so be prepared to undress the infant. Have a blanket to wrap the child in, as well as extra diapers/wipes, and a bottle just in case you have a wait (that's why it's called the waiting room). If you wish to minimize your wait time, schedule your appointment for the first thing in the morning (9, 9:15 or 9:30) or right after lunch (1:15, 1:30, 1:45). Wait times tend to be shorter at the beginning of each session and your infant will be exposed to fewer sick contacts at those times. As the morning or afternoon progresses there is an increased risk that your provider will fall behind on the schedule. This is not planned, but emergencies come up which can set the schedule awry. Older children appreciate a few books or toys to pass the time. A few snacks in a baggie can be a life saver. Bring in a notebook with your questions written ahead of time. Be aware that most providers have around 10 to 15 minutes for each patient, so things will move quickly. Ask your questions as soon as possible (at the beginning of the visit), to give the provider time to address any concerns. Jot answers down, to help remember them later. Studies show that parents retain only about 10% of what providers tell them. If possible, ask your healthcare provider to give you handouts with the baby's height and weight, with percentages.

Growth chart

In a well exam, the first thing we do is check the height, weight, and head circumference (size of the head) on something called a growth chart. Babies are compared in two ways: in comparison to other babies their own age as well as in comparison to their previous visits. This curve is expressed in percentages: 3%, 5%, 10%, 25%, 50%, 75%, 90%, 95%, and 97%. There is not one good and one bad percentage. You may be told that your baby is at the 50% for height: that means your baby is average compared to other same sex babies the same age. It's not so much the percentage, but the comparison to the previous percentage that's important. We expect the baby to follow a track (it's a path) on a growth curve. If your child was at the 75% for weight at the last visit and now is at the 5% for weight, that's a concern due to the large change. It's the large changes in percentage that we watch. I would then address feeding issues, after I rechecked the weight.

If you ask your healthcare provider, they will show the growth chart to you. Many babies are either above or below average. Neither is a problem, but we watch for large changes from the baby's normal growth patterns. If any issues are found, your healthcare provider will discuss this with you. Don't be afraid to ask to see the growth chart for height, weight, and head circumference. Write it down and keep track of it. We compare these percentages at each well visit to be sure that your child is growing as expected. With the new EMR's (Electronic Medical Records) the growth charts are stored in the computer. This way they can be reviewed at each well visit. If your healthcare provider is not showing you the growth chart during your child's well exam, please ask them to do so. If you don't understand them, ask questions. After all, this is your child, and you need to understand how they are growing. Be aware that growth charts are generally not reviewed during sick visits.

Immunizations

The well exam is also an important time for immunizations. Immunizations are given at most check-ups as a routine part of the visit. Many parents ask questions about immunizations. First, it is absolutely normal for you to be concerned about what is placed into your infant's body. Secondly, it is vitally important that you understand that the vaccines are based on YEARS of scientific research. There are few things that anger me more than a website or group of persons who denounce vaccines without scientific fact. We must understand that vaccines are tested, safe, effective, and reliable. They offer protection from deadly diseases. The vaccine schedule is determined by the Center for Disease Control (CDC) and approved by the American Academy of Pediatrics (AAP). This schedule is routinely updated.

My mother was born in 1922. She used to tell me how afraid they were of diseases like polio. In fact, one of my cousins was permanently crippled by polio. Mom wondered if it was safe to send her children to school or take them to the market or church. She was so relieved when the polio vaccine was developed. She rushed to the medical office to get her children immunized so that they wouldn't have to face that dreaded disease. They stood in line for hours to get vaccinated.

Today, I feel like I work to convince more and more concerned families that they should immunize their children. Facts prove that it is FAR SAFER to immunize than not. Parents today have never seen or heard of most of these diseases. There is little or no fear of them. I agree, fear should not affect our decisions, but fear is the tool anti-vaccine websites use to influence parents not to vaccinate. By NOT vaccinating, one takes on the risk of disease, so both vaccinating and not vaccinating carry risk. Everything has risk, even driving in a car, yet we all do that daily. These diseases do still exist. They can sicken or even kill your child. Vaccines are safe and effective in preventing deadly diseases.

Autism

Well, I can't speak about vaccines without discussing the tragedy of the myth about autism and vaccines. As I am sure you are aware, there was media hype about autism being caused by vaccines, specifically the MMR: Measles, Mumps, and Rubella vaccine. Although this myth has been dispelled scientifically over and over, it perpetuates. It began in 1998, when a British physician, Andrew Wakefield, made claims about vaccines causing autism. His unfounded suggestions caused a decrease in the number of children who received vaccines, particularly the MMR. This decrease in vaccination may have contributed to the increase in measles. His ideas were scientifically disproven, and he fell into professional disrepute. He stopped practicing medicine in 2004 and has been disbarred by the British Medical Council. In summary, vaccines do not cause autism, and never did. The truth is, we don't really know what exactly causes autism, but we have been able to prove that it's not vaccines. We now believe that autism may have a more genetic role. The definition of autism keeps changing, and that's why you see some fluctuation in the numbers of children with autism. Bottom line: vaccines don't cause autism…vaccines prevent diseases.

Never-the less, most parents understand the value of vaccines. They prevent disease. They are tested and safe. It usually takes 10 years or more to develop a vaccine. Why? Because vaccines must be proven AND effective prior to release. They MUST be tested. Most vaccines work by tricking the body into thinking it has been attacked by disease so that it will develop specific antibodies (our body's defense) against that disease. It is these antibodies that will later protect us against any exposure to that disease.

Vaccines are given on a timed schedule for a reason, to protect the child during periods of time when the child is the most susceptible to a disease. When the vaccines are administered is important, as the recommended vaccine schedule has been studied and shown to coordinate with the child's immune system to provide protection at the time when the child is at the highest risk for a certain disease. Some vaccines need booster doses (multiple doses of a certain vaccine) due to the length of time that the vaccine offers protection. Spacing vaccines is NOT recommended as it may leave an infant or child vulnerable to a disease for a longer period. I do not recommend an altered vaccine schedule. Giving vaccines on an altered schedule can put a child at risk. Concern regarding overwhelming the child's immune system with multiple vaccines is unwarranted as children are exposed to more germs daily (just through normal life) than through the recommended vaccines. I recommend following the recommended vaccine schedule and vaccinating ON TIME for the best protection against deadly diseases.

Believe me, these diseases still exist. These diseases are deadly. We need to protect our precious children against these deadly diseases. The best way to protect your child is to give your child the vaccines in the series recommended by the CDC (Center for Disease Control). My kids are protected…are yours?

The vaccines that are given to children include:

- **DTaP** which protects against diphtheria, tetanus and pertussis (whooping cough). These are deadly diseases. It is given in five doses at ages 2 months, 4 months, 6 months, 15 to 18 months, and age 4 to 6 years.
- **MMR*** which protects against measles, mumps and rubella (German measles). It is given in two doses at age 12 to 15 months and 4 to 6 years.
- **IPV** which protects against polio, a disease which can cripple. It is given in four doses at 2, 4, and 6 to 18 months, and 4 to 6 years.
- **Hib** which protects against Hemophilus influenze type b, which can cause meningitis. It is given in three or four doses at 2, 4, and 6 months, then at 12 to 15 months.

- **Hep A** which protects against Hepatitis A, a liver disease passed through eating food. It is given in two doses 6 months apart, starting at 12 to 23 months.
- **Hep B** which protects against Hepatitis B, a liver disease. It is given in three doses at birth, 1 to 2 months, and 6 to 18 months.
- **Varicella*** which protects against the chickenpox virus. It is given in two doses at 12 to 15 months, and 4 to 6 years.
- **Tdap** which protects against tetanus, diphtheria, and pertussis for older children and adults. It is given between 11 to 12 years. (Most children get this prior to middle school).
- **PCV** which protects against bacterial meningitis, pneumonia and bloodstream infections. It also offers some protection against ear infections. It is given in four doses at 2, 4, 6 months and 12 to 15 months.
- **MCV-4** which protects against four types of meningococcal disease (serogroups A, C, W and Y), a disease of the layering of the brain. This disease can be lethal. It is given in two doses at 11 to 12 years and 16 years.
- **Men-B** which protects against Serogroup B Meningococcal Vaccines. It is given to high risk children at 16 years and 18 years.

- **Rota*** which protects against rotavirus, an intestinal virus which causes severe diarrhea. It is given in two or three doses to infants at 2, 4, and 6 months.
- **HPV** which protects against the human papilloma virus. This virus can cause cervical cancer in women and oral cancers in men. If given between 11 and 15 years of age, two doses are adequate when given six months apart. If given after 15 years of age, three doses are required: dose two is 2 months after dose one, and dose three is 6 months after dose one.
- **Flu** protects against certain strains of influenza. It is strongly recommended annually in the early fall for all children and infants over six months of age.
- These schedules are revised routinely. Changes will be updated by your healthcare provider.

    *indicates live virus vaccines

You can be assured that every vaccine is tested and sampled. All additives are disclosed. There are four stages of clinical testing. The testing takes years, and lots of volunteers, who receive the vaccine. The vaccines are studied and the Food and Drug Administration (FDA) reviews everything:

the trial results, product labeling, safety, and side effects. Therefore, you can rest assured that the vaccines are safe.

The bare bones **TRUTH** of the matter is that children are far more likely to be harmed by serious infectious disease than by immunizations. Most side effects are local and include redness, swelling and soreness. There may be mild fever for 24 hours with some vaccines. If your child has fever or fussiness after a vaccine, then give them Children's Tylenol (acetaminophen) based on their weight, no more often than every four hours. If they are not fussy or feverish, then they don't need any medication. The initial reaction of fever is helpful to the body to start developing the immunity to the disease. I do not recommend giving your child Tylenol prior to vaccination.

Do I vaccinate my children? YES! I've done the research. I've read the data. I very much believe in vaccinating. I try to respect others wishes but do your own research and draw your own conclusions. Be sure to check SCIENTIFICALLY validated FACTS!

Here are some credible websites you may wish to reference:

www.cdc.gov/vaccines/

www.immunize.org

Developmental Milestones

Finally at the routine well visit, we watch for the all-important developmental milestones to assure us that your child is developing appropriately (to be sure that they are doing what they should be doing at each age). There is some normal variance child to child, so be careful about comparing your child to a neighbor's child or a sibling. If your healthcare provider notices a delay in development, don't panic. Some children just take longer to do certain things. If delays persist for more than one visit, your provider may recommend additional evaluation, perhaps with a neurodevelopmental pediatrician, or maybe some physical therapy.

Newborn

A newborn baby does little more than cry, but should move their arms and legs. They will try to pick their little head off of your shoulder. They may be wobbly but will hold their head up for a few moments. You will notice that they will wrap their little fingers around one of yours and hold on. They should gaze into your eyes as you feed them. They may follow your gaze if you move your head. It's important to hold a baby to feed them, so even if you bottle feed, please don't prop the bottle. The infant needs your touch and interaction to thrive. They need to associate that safe warm feeling of being fed with being in a loving parent's arms. You will notice that the baby will startle if there is a loud noise like a door slamming. A baby may squint to a bright sunny day. This all reassures us that the baby can see and hear and move.

Two months

By two months old the baby may start to roll from his/her belly to his/her back. Be careful, they can roll off of things and get hurt. Yes, the baby should be sleeping on the back, but needs supervised tummy time when awake. Practice rolling by playing with the baby on the floor. Gently roll the baby back and forth (belly to back), protecting the head. Toys are not as important as the time spent with you. Many two-month-olds don't roll, as they may not get enough tummy time. You can work on this. We have gotten away from just playing with kids. I saw a baby in the mall last week watching an IPAD. Our infants don't need electronics; they need us. Avoid use of technology (except video chatting with Grandma) in children less than 18 months of age. Just sitting on the floor and interacting is important. This is vital to your child's development, both physically and intellectually. A two month old should be able to swat at objects in front of them. They coo and make adorable baby noises. You get mostly vowel sounds like "oooohhhh".

They may make noises in response to you speaking to them. They are learning the timing of conversation. You speak, and then they speak. They have a social smile in response to yours. They show particular pleasure in seeing their parents. While lying on the stomach, they can lift their head, neck, and upper chest while supporting their weight on their forearms.

Four months

At four months, babies babble and coo. You will likely hear the delightful sound of a baby's laughter. There is not a better sound in the world. They may squeal, which may thrill or frighten them. On the stomach (only while awake) they can support the weight of their upper body on their hands. They will hold a rattle, and reach for objects. They will roll from tummy to back, as well as from back to tummy. Again, many four-month-olds may not roll if they are not getting AWAKE, supervised tummy time. Always remember to sleep on the back to decrease the risk of sudden infant death (SIDS). This age has better head control when held. They will turn to a noise, and recognize their parent's voices.

Six months

By six months old, babies are really fun. They can sit with support for a short period of time. Be careful, as they will still fall over if left unattended, so practice sitting while on the ground, surrounded by pillows. They babble in response to your speech. They will stand when placed in that position and can hold their weight with your support. They recognize their parents. They can transfer an object (like a block or rattle) from one hand to the other hand. Of course, everything goes in the mouth, so be cautious. Babies should not play with items that are small enough to pass through a toilet paper roll, as they may be choking hazards. They can easily roll. Do not leave them near stairs, as they may roll and fall. They will pick up small items off the floor and place them in their mouth. Again, be careful with choking hazards. If you have an older child with Legos, beware. This is a great time to baby proof the house. I recommend that you sit on the floor and see what babies can get into. Cover any outlets and pad sharp edges of furniture. Secure loose cords. Move cleaning supplies and chemicals upward. Secure cabinets with baby safe locks. Safety first.

Nine months

Nine months is my favorite age. They respond to their name. They understand some words. They babble mamma, dadddda. They may crawl, but not all babies do. Some scoot. Some army crawl. They poke things with their finger. They love the "drop it so mommy can pick it up" game. (I hate that game.) They love peek-a-boo and patty cake. They will pick up food and feed themselves. They will grasp a Cheerio with their thumb and index (pointer) finger. This is called a pincher grasp. They may be afraid of strangers, but will delight in their parents. They pull up to a stand in the crib. They raise their arms to be picked up. They are cherubs.

Twelve months

At twelve months, they will say between two and four words, usually "dada" (for daddy), "mama" (for mommy), and maybe one other word. Don't expect too much vocabulary just yet. They will hold on and walk around the crib or the coffee table, and may stand independently for a moment before plopping down to the ground. They can drink from a cup and wave bye-bye. They prefer to feed themselves. They look for dropped or hidden objects. This is called object permanence. The child now knows that the object still exists even if he/she cannot see it. They are no longer an infant, now a child. (Time to start planning for a little brother or sister?)

Age Appropriate Anticipatory Guidance

At each well visit, your healthcare provider should go over age appropriate anticipatory guidance for your child. Anticipatory guidance are safety measures that will be appropriate for your child's age. These items should vary at each visit, and be directed at the child's age. For example at the three to five day visit you will be reminded that an infant needs to sleep on their back (and pacifiers may help) to decrease the risk of Sudden Infant Death Syndrome (SIDS). The car seat needs to be backward facing until two years of age. The water heater should be set not higher than 120 degrees F to avoid scalding burns. Babies are most often injured by burns or falls, so use caution around hot liquids including coffee. Do not cook holding your baby. Do not leave a baby unattended on any surface, as they may fall. Do not put a baby to bed with a bottle, as they can get baby bottle tooth decay. They may discuss child-proofing the home, especially as the baby becomes more active. The use of baby walkers is discouraged due to the risk of falls, particularly down stairs. Baby's teeth can be brushed with water as soon as they have teeth. The first dental visit is now encouraged at 12 months of age. Check to see if your water contains fluoride. Fluoride is protective for teeth. The use of screen time (other than video chatting with grandma) is strongly discouraged in children less than 18 months old. These discussions help prepare the parent to have a safe environment for the child.

Closing the visit

At the end of each visit, you should be reminded when to return for the next well examination. They should offer to schedule that visit as you leave if possible, and give you a reminder card, as well as a reminder phone call, email, or text prior to the visit. You should be asked if you have any other questions or concerns, as well as if you understood what was discussed during the visit. I'm sure you are aware that healthcare providers are on a strict time schedule, but your time is valuable as well. Review your notebook, did you get all your questions answered? Write down the next visit, and be sure to get the after-hours or emergency phone number just in case. This is also a great time to review if the office has evening or Saturday hours for such emergencies. You should always know how to reach the on-call provider for any middle-of-the-night emergencies.

In this chapter, we have covered what is discussed in the well visit which should occur at 2 weeks, 2, 4, 6, 9, 12, 15, 18, 24, 30, and 36 months. As I have stressed, the well checkup is crucial for the child's well-being. Schedule your child's next well visit today.

Sick visits

What about your sick child? Sick visits are made as needed. Sick visits do not replace well visits, so just because your child got sick at six months, doesn't mean that you don't need a six month well visit. Sick visits only deal with the illness at hand. At our office, approximately 50% of our daily schedule is held open for same day sick appointments. You should be able to get your child into your provider the same day you call if your child is ill. Children get sick fast and need to be evaluated quickly. If you have a health related question, you should be able to speak to a triage nurse relatively quickly, and you should be able to be seen the same day. If you routinely have to wait more than a day to get a sick appointment, look for another provider or another pediatric practice.

Sick babies under two months of age

Any illness in a child less than two months old should be evaluated as soon as possible. If a child less than 60 days old has a fever (rectal temperature greater than 100.4 degrees F), they will need to go to an office or a hospital for an evaluation immediately. If you're not sure of the temperature, but you think it's around 100 degrees F, don't risk it. Take the baby to a healthcare provider. This is urgent. You should also take a child under two months old to a healthcare provider if they have a cough or runny nose, rash, vomiting or diarrhea, fever or fussiness. At this age, any symptom should be evaluated, as very young children are more vulnerable to disease.

Fever

Believe it or not, fever is our friend. Fever lets us parents know that our children are ill. Fever raises the body temperature in order to attempt to eradicate the offending disease process. Fevers are much more common in children older than 30 days. Most medical literature defines a fever as a rectal temperature at or above 100.4 degrees F (38 degrees C). A rectal temperature is the most accurate temperature. Of course children get colds, but a runny nose or cough that persists longer than a week should always be evaluated. A fever that persists more than three days should be evaluated, as well as **any fever in a child less than two months of age**. Fever in an infant less than 2 months of age requires **immediate** medical evaluation. Fever that occurs (in children older than 2 months) later in the illness (not the first few days) should be evaluated. Vomiting and diarrhea, fussiness or sleeplessness, rashes, change in appetite or behavior are all signs that should be evaluated by a healthcare provider. Trust your parental instinct. If you have a feeling that something is just not quite right, it's better to play it safe and get things checked out. It's better to err on the side of caution. Children get different illnesses than adults and should be evaluated promptly. They get well quickly, but can also get seriously ill very quickly. This book is not intended to replace the advice of your healthcare provider. Always follow recommendations given by your healthcare provider.

Colds

There are more than 200 strains of cold viruses. Children will get colds. They will have runny noses. Most colds, or upper respiratory infections, last about a week to 10 days. Children usually get their first cold after six months of age, but it can occur at a younger age. Colds are more frequent in those children attending daycare, as they have more exposure to other children. Children can get up to 20 colds in a year, so you can understand that it may seem like a young child always has a runny nose. I always tell parents to circle healthy days on the calendar so that we can tell how long they are sick between well days. Sometimes a child may have only two or three well days between illnesses. Any illness lasting longer than a week should be evaluated. Any fever lasting longer than three days should be evaluated (or any fever in an infant less than two months should be evaluated immediately). You can help the symptoms of a cold by offering children's Tylenol (dosed based on weight rather than age) to a fussy or feverish baby older than two months. Running a cool mist humidifier may be helpful as well. Be sure to clean your humidifier frequently to prevent mold growth. No cough or cold medications are recommended for children under four years of age. You can, however, use nasal saline spray and bulb suction the child's nose, particularly prior to feedings. It sometimes helps to slightly elevate the head of the infant's bed by placing a blanket underneath the mattress, but be careful not to have too steep of an incline or the baby will roll to the bottom. Sometimes nursing a baby while sitting in a steamy bathroom can help open a stuffy nose. I also recommend frequent feeds, since babies don't drink or nurse as well when their nose is plugged.

Stomach virus

The common stomach virus, or acute gastroenteritis, is characterized by a rapid onset of recurrent vomiting which may go on for a day or two, followed by loose stools (diarrhea) which may go on for up to two weeks. You must be careful to avoid dehydration with these types of illnesses. With stomach bugs, it's best to avoid milk products, Motrin, and citrus juices for at least the first day. I usually will put young infants on Pedialyte for no more than six eight hours, and then return the baby to breast milk or formula. Watch for signs of dehydration including lack of wetting for more than six hours, dry cracked lips, and extreme fatigue. If you are concerned that your sick baby may be dehydrated, have the child evaluated immediately at the pediatric office or local emergency department.

Rashes

Rashes were discussed briefly in Chapter 5, but the subject bears mention here. Most viral rashes begin with fever first, then the fever goes away. The next day or so, the rash appears. There are many viral rashes including roseola, hand, foot, and mouth, and fifths disease. Since these rashes are viral, no treatment is needed. I do not recommend creams or lotions for viral rashes as they will resolve on their own without treatment. Not all rashes are viral, however, which is why I will recommend that you see your pediatric healthcare provider if your child gets a rash. If it is a viral rash, your child is usually no longer contagious after the rash develops, so they can generally return to daycare. Always consult your pediatric healthcare provider to be sure.

Bacterial vs. viral illnesses

Some illnesses, such as colds, are viral. They will not respond to antibiotics and generally go away without treatment in about a week to 10 days. Some illnesses are caused by bacteria, such as urinary tract infections, and need to be treated with antibiotics. Sometimes there is pressure from parents to ask providers for antibiotics to treat viruses. Unfortunately, antibiotics do not cure viruses, but because viruses pass on their own, the parents think that the antibiotics helped. This misuse of antibiotics is causing a problem known as antibiotic resistance. When we need the antibiotics to work, they may not, as the germs are becoming more and more resistant to the overused antibiotics. This is not to say that you shouldn't use an antibiotic when it is recommended by your healthcare provider. You certainly should. I would just like to caution that if it is viral, and your healthcare provider verifies that it is viral, then an antibiotic is not necessary or recommended.

Antibiotics

If your child has a bacterial infection, such as a sinus infection, ear infection or urinary tract infection, then your healthcare provider will prescribe an antibiotic for your child. Always complete the full course of antibiotic and follow up as directed. Your child may seem better after a few days, but it is very important to complete the full course of antibiotics, as the infection may recur if you do not. It can be dangerous to only partially treat an infection, so always finish the full course of antibiotics. I recommend giving your child a probiotic with the antibiotic. The probiotic contains healthy bacteria that is found in the gut. This helps to replace normal intestinal flora, as the antibiotic may upset the natural balance in the intestine. Many infant formulas contain probiotics, so if your child's formula contains probiotics, then you do not need to add an additional probiotic. Your healthcare provider can advise you whether to add a probiotic.

Coughing

Coughing babies should be evaluated by their healthcare provider. Particularly young infants are at higher risk for diseases of cough, including pertussis (the whooping cough or the 100-day-cough), RSV (Respiratory Syncytial Virus), and bronchiolitis. If your child is coughing, watch for color change with cough. This should be evaluated immediately if the child is in respiratory distress or is turning blue (dial 911). If you hear wheezing, very rapid breathing, or see your child's chest pulling in, seek immediate medical care. These respiratory illnesses often require medical intervention.

Cold sores

I need to stress the seriousness of cold sores in parents. Cold sores are blisters that occur on the edge of lip. Before the blisters erupt, you may feel a tingling or burning sensation. They are caused by the herpes simplex virus (HSV). There are two strains of HSV. Cold sores are typically caused by HSV-1. This virus is very contagious and spreads by skin-to-skin contact. Cold sores may seem like a minor irritation to us adults, but they can be extremely dangerous, even deadly, to a new infant. This can cause severe infection in a newborn or young infant. About 1 in 3,500 infants born in the

U.S. get neonatal herpes. Some cases occur from exposure during birth and some cases from exposure after birth. If you have a cold sore, DO NOT KISS your baby until the sore has completely healed. Do everything you can to limit the baby's exposure to the cold sore: keeping it covered (if possible), no kissing, and frequent hand washing. Be sure to advise other adults that may be holding or handling your baby not to kiss the baby if they have a cold sore (or feel one starting). It is possible to have cold sores and not spread them to your family. If you have concerns that your infant has HSV, contact your pediatric healthcare provider.

When can my sick baby return to daycare?

The policy of most daycare institutions is to send babies home who have a fever or other contagious illness. The children are usually considered contagious until they have been fever-free (off Tylenol or Motrin) for 24 hours. They can then return to daycare. If you are not sure if your child should return to daycare, you can consult with your pediatric healthcare provider, as well as the policy of your daycare.

Summary

Whether sick, or well, children need specialized healthcare. They need routine well examinations to check their growth and development. They need prompt sick care. You, as a parent, have a right to quality pediatric healthcare that is explained to you in a way that you can understand. Always feel free to ask questions, and ask again if you feel you did not get your question answered or if you do not understand. If you are not satisfied with the care you are receiving, make changes in your provider. Check with your insurance company to view other providers in the area that are covered under your plan. Make visits, speak to the parents in the waiting room, speak to the front desk help, question the nurses, and meet with the providers. Find a practice that meets your needs for scheduling, location, and philosophy. You will be working with this group of providers for 20 years, so you will want a good fit. Please don't forget to keep up with those well examinations.

Key points:

- Well visits are important to observe growth and development.
- Certified Pediatric Nurse Practitioners and Board Certified Pediatricians specialize in the care of children.
- Prepare for doctor visits; bring your questions written out.
- Compare the growth curves to the previous growth curve.
- Immunizations are tested, safe, effective, and reliable.
- Vaccines do not cause autism.
- Diseases are deadly, vaccines are safe.
- Developmental milestones help to assure appropriate development.
- Anticipatory guidance is offered at visits to address safety concerns.
- Don't kiss your baby if you have a cold sore.
- Sick children need prompt evaluation.

Raising Today's Baby

Raising Today's Baby

Chapter 7: Feeding time again?

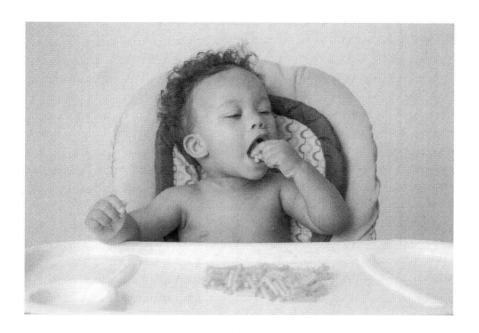

Raising Today's Baby

Chapter 7: Feeding time again?

Of course, we all know what babies eat. But what is best: breast or bottle? How much? How often? Parents, who want to do everything right, are often confused by the many choices available. This topic is timely and pervasive; it's the stuff of endless media coverage and debate. This chapter will discuss the latest recommendations, and as always, I advise that you discuss these topics with your healthcare provider to help you make the best decisions for your family.

When our first child was born, I was young and inexperienced. I had worked in pediatric nursing at a children's hospital, but it was different with my own baby. I was broke, as I had delivered him between jobs, and had no health insurance. I had college loans to pay off as well. So not only did I have a new infant, I had a big hospital bill.

My husband and I were both working full-time, just to get by. I remember buying a loaf of bread and a jar of peanut butter, and that was all we had to eat for that entire week. Of course, my child had formula and diapers. We chose to go without eating meat or dining out, so our son would not have to do without. Isn't that true of all mothers and caregivers? Our children are dressed like mini movie stars, but we wear our shoes until they fall apart. Sacrificing for one's child is a universal trait, and indicative of the selfless love we feel as parents.

So, as I was facing the decision of what to feed my child, getting back to work was absolutely essential to survival. I was exhausted from delivering a nearly 10-pound baby. You can imagine I was not feeling well. I briefly considered breastfeeding, but with little encouragement, physical exhaustion, a short maternity leave (four weeks), and a post-delivery infection, I decided to formula feed my son. I never even tried breastfeeding. It was a decision I later regretted.

I had better success breastfeeding my daughter. I had a lovely experience with her. I now try to encourage my patients to breastfeed whenever it is possible. Most mothers can successfully breastfeed. You need to understand that these are personal decisions, and ultimately each parent must make the right decision for their personal situation. I am here to share information and support, as well as my own struggles, both truthfully and professionally as a caring mother and healthcare provider.

I know full well, and understand what it's like, both as a parent and a healthcare professional, to go through difficult times. I do not believe that we should judge what others choose to do, even when we staunchly disagree with their methods, as we may not fully understand their circumstances. When I was starting out, though I knew, professionally speaking, that breast was best, my personal and financial standing still determined my choice to bottle feed.

Helpful facts:

- Newborns normally take one to two ounces every two to two and a half hours if they are bottle fed. An average sized infant will drink one to two ounces easily. Breastfed newborns generally eat a bit more often at first, perhaps even nursing every hour and a half to two hours initially. Newborns need to be fed AT LEAST every three hours around the clock, which is especially important for the first two weeks, until the baby is back to birth weight. Most babies lose some weight after birth, which is generally regained by two weeks of age. The first two weeks is a crucial period, because babies can dehydrate quickly. When they get dehydrated, they become weak, so they don't feed as vigorously, leading to further dehydration, and further weakness. This can be serious or even critical if the weight loss exceeds 10% of their birth weight. Therefore, it's vital to see your healthcare provider at between three to five days of life and within 48 to 72 hours of discharge from the hospital. The next visit will come at two weeks of life.

- Babies from one month to four months gradually increase their feeds from four to six ounces, continuing to want to feed about every three hours around the clock. The nighttime feeds naturally begin to space themselves to every four to five hours, but not for all babies.

- After four months, most babies eat about six to eight ounces every three to four hours around the clock. Sometimes these babies will space their nighttime feeds to every five to six hours. During periods of growth, you may notice your baby waking to feed more frequently again. Babies have week-long growth spurts that occur at around 2, 6, and 12 weeks of life. You may notice that your child is hungry and wanting to feed more frequently during these times.

When will my baby sleep through the night?

Babies usually need to eat every three to four hours through the night. The age at which a baby will sleep through the night varies but is usually between five and six months of age. Most texts define "sleeping through the night" as between midnight and five a.m. That certainly would not be MY definition of sleeping through the night. I want to sleep from 10 p.m. until at least 6 a.m. Some babies will "sleep through" the night sooner than six months, however, I am very tolerant of nighttime feedings through the age of nine months. After nine months, if your child's weight is good, it is likely not necessary for your child to feed at night. Sometimes breastfed children will continue to nurse at night. Due to the very rapid growth babies younger than six months are experiencing, it is necessary for them to feed through the night to keep up with the caloric demand placed upon their developing bodies.

After nine months, a healthy sized baby does not need to be fed during the night. This doesn't mean that they still won't ask for it! It means that they can be comforted and encouraged to go back to sleep without a bottle or breast. My children were different from one another when it came to night sleeping. My son, the big eater, slept through by around six months. My daughter, who is still tiny, would continue to wake through until about three years of age. After nine months, you can get something called "trained wakening." The kids wake up because they always have, and if you go in to give them a drink, you reinforce that wakening. I was guilty of this with my daughter, because at that time I was working during the day and three a.m. became our private play time. I can honestly say I don't regret a minute of that middle-of-the-night party time, as those were magic moments together. I must add, however, that it was positively exhausting. A friend of mine, who is a Certified Lactation Consultant, does recommend continued nighttime feedings for breastfeeding moms if it is working for both mom and baby.

How do I know my baby is getting enough formula/breast milk?

I am frequently asked this question. The answer is simple enough. You can tell if a newborn is getting enough formula/breast milk if:

1. Your baby (over one week of age) is producing at least six wet diapers in a 24-hour period, with one diaper being soaking wet. (Younger infants will need to be weighed and evaluated in the office.)

2. Your baby is stooling several times daily.

3. Your healthcare provider documents adequate weight gain. (This is usually discussed at the visit at three days of life, two weeks, and then two months.) The goal is to regain weight back to birth weight by the two-week visit, then to maintain a steady track on the growth chart. Ask your healthcare provider to show you the growth chart for comparison. The growth chart shows your baby in comparison to other babies, as well as in relation to their previous height and weight.

What is the growth chart?

At each well visit, your healthcare provider should give you statistics in percentages for height, weight, and head circumference. These compare your baby to other babies of the same age, as well as comparing your baby to themselves at a younger age. For example, if your child's height is in the 90th percentile, he or she is taller than 90% of children of the same sex and age. The 50th percentile would be average. Just because a child may be below average on height or weight is not necessarily cause for worry. As is the case with adults, babies come in all shapes and sizes. Some are taller, and some are smaller. What *is* important is to watch the trend over time to be sure that your child continues to grow and gain weight.

Important Tip: Dehydration

If you have concerns that your newborn is NOT getting enough formula/breast milk, call your healthcare provider today. Do not wait. The first two weeks are a critical time. This is especially true if your infant is difficult to wake and is not producing six wet diapers (one being soaked) in a 24-hour period. Newborns may not make six diapers the first few days, but I would expect six wet diapers per day by six days of age. Watch for signs of dehydration which can be serious, even life-threatening, if not addressed quickly. These include increased sleepiness, poor feeding effort, weight loss, and not enough wet diapers. When new parents tell me that the baby is "so good" or doesn't want to wake to feed, I feel concern. These can be signs of dehydration in a newborn. Seek immediate medical care if you have concerns that your baby may be dehydrated as this can be life-threatening in infants.

Burping

OK, I fed the baby, now what? Sure, everyone knows that babies need to be burped! Well if that's true, why do I spend so many afternoons helping new parents with this task? The reason is that it's not always as easy as it looks. To an "experienced mom," burping may be everyday stuff, but to a new mom or dad, it can be a frightening and impossible task. We tend to get a little impatient. We're all sleep-deprived anyway, and when burping doesn't occur quickly, we give up and move on. This can leave a baby very uncomfortable and gassy. Babies, like most of us, need to burp after sucking and swallowing air. This air can then cause the infant considerable gas pain in their stomachs, which leads to crying and fussiness. This happens more often to babies than to adults, since we are experienced eaters and swallow less air than they do. Other mammals, including cows, also burp. In some animals, an inability to burp can be fatal, a condition called bloat. I feel like this after every Thanksgiving dinner. In the case of bloat, a vet needs to place a tube into the esophagus to relieve the pressure. I've never heard of a fatal case of gas in an infant, but it sure can kill a good night's sleep.

When I ask new parents if the baby is difficult to burp, most of them say, "YES!" Now, I doubt that nearly all the babies that I see in the office are difficult to burp. What I suspect is that the parents are unsure of the correct technique required to actually obtain a burp. I was lucky, as I grew up babysitting, and then worked as a pediatric nurse at a children's hospital. On our hospital floor, we cared only for infants between the ages of birth and 12 months. They had to be fed every three hours, and we cared for between three and six babies a shift. That's up to 18 feedings per 8-hour shift. This was how I learned to feed and burp infants. Of course, besides feeding, we had to give medications and baths, do dressing changes, hand IVs, and monitor vital signs. It was a busy job, indeed, but one which taught me a great deal about babies, as well as organizational skills.

Why do babies need to be burped right after feeding?

When they drink, they gulp air with the milk and swallow it. If they are not burped, the air will just travel through the digestive system and come out as gas…eventually. It also will make their little tummies hurt, and when babies hurt, they cry. When babies cry, moms feed them. Without a good burp, more gas goes through and you get the picture… more crying. It's a dreadful cycle. By the time I see them in the office, everyone is upset! Oftentimes, BOTH mom and baby are crying. This often can be prevented by a good burp. So how do I burp a baby? Well, I recommend one burp in the middle of the feed, after one breast, or after one ounce in a newborn, and the second burp at the end of the feed. Be sure to take your time; sometimes it takes several minutes to properly burp a baby.

The most common error in burping that I see is incorrect technique. People generally gently pat or rub a baby on the back. Of course, we need to be gentle. We never want to hurt a baby and NEVER want to shake a baby. Shaking a baby can cause SHAKEN BABY SYNDROME, resulting in brain damage and even death.

Using a cupped hand (the cupped hand is VITAL) and bending at the wrist, gently but FIRMLY and SLOWLY burp the baby. If dads are unsure about how much force to use, I recommend that they use their non-dominant hand (if you are right handed, use your left hand). Be sure to hold the baby securely, especially the head. Place the baby on your shoulder or sitting in your lap. Remember to use the motion in your wrist. Continue burping until you hear a nice burp. I usually tell people to practice the technique on their thighs. If you pat your thigh gently, notice how your fat doesn't jiggle, but if you "burp" your thigh with the cupped hand and adequate firmness, the fat on your thigh should jiggle a little. Notice that it doesn't hurt to hit your thigh with a cupped hand, since that catches air and cushions the blow. Never burp a baby with a bare back. Burping should never leave a mark…enough said.

I have been asked if all babies burp. I try to avoid words like *all* or *never*, as there are always exceptions. Babies do not read textbooks. I would answer that most babies burp. I can usually get a baby to burp. I believe it helps babies to feel more comfortable and is important in that aspect.

Important Tip: Never Shake a Baby

Never shake a baby. This can result in Shaken Baby Syndrome and leads to extreme brain damage and even death. It doesn't take much force to cause Shaken Baby Syndrome. If you are frustrated with your baby, put him/her in the crib (side rails up) on their back for safety, and then walk away. Just take a few moments to compose yourself before returning to care for the child. A mug of herbal tea in your favorite chair may help you to calm down.

Formula vs. Breastfeeding

Of course, it's no secret that breast is best. It is nature's perfect food. It's free, warm, already prepared and packaged, and, portable. Most mothers can successfully breastfeed with support and encouragement. With my son, sadly, I didn't breastfeed, as I headed almost immediately back to work. I was ill and tired and unable to handle one more thing. Although I knew breastfeeding was the better option, I chose to go the "simple route" and give formula. To be fair, there was not a great deal of support for breastfeeding during that time. Afterwards, I regretted that decision. I felt like I missed an opportunity to give my child important maternal antibodies, and indeed my son had many ear infections. My son gained weight faster than my daughter and continues to struggle with weight issues. There is some discussion that formula-fed infants have higher levels of insulin due to the high protein of formula. Higher insulin levels are associated with weight gain and obesity. It is thought that breastfeeding can decrease a child's risk for obesity. It is believed that the longer the child is nursed, the lower the risk of obesity.

When I had my daughter six years later, it was a different story. I was older and more prepared. I had done my research and not only wanted to breastfeed but loved the experience! My milk production was not what it should have been, so I had to do some supplementation with formula, but I was blessed to have the time to nurture my child.

Even if you can only breastfeed for a short time, I would encourage you to try. You give your baby immunity through the milk, which helps prevent illnesses and infections. Also breast-fed infants tend to regulate their internal cues for hunger better than formula-fed infants because of Leptin, the hormone which regulates appetite. Breast-fed infants are at a lower risk for obesity. My daughter has never once struggled with weight. Now, whether that is due to genetic or other factors, such as breastfeeding, who knows? Breastfeeding is also such a personal bonding experience. I cherish the time we had together during this special season of life. I think my daughter and I have always been close because of it. If you are like me, and don't make enough milk, there are things which you can do to stimulate milk production, or you can supplement (as I did) with some formula. I strongly recommend breastfeeding whenever possible. Breast is best.

Breastfeeding

As I already stated, healthcare providers recommend breastfeeding as the best option. It is pre-packaged, always ready, inexpensive, pre-warmed, and nutritionally sound. It is in-fact nature's way. But, many new moms and newborns have some degree of difficulty during breastfeeding. There are many complete texts on this subject alone. If you are having difficulty breastfeeding, please consult your pediatric healthcare provider, a Certified Lactation Consultant (www.ilca.org), or the La Leche League (www.llli.org). Sometimes an experienced breastfeeding mom can offer some helpful insights and tips.

Most breastfeeding difficulties occur in the first month of breastfeeding, especially within the first few weeks. Often it is a combination of fatigue, post-partum depression, and sore nipples which cause discouragement with the process. Don't give up. Most moms can successfully breastfeed.

Here are a few tips to help:

1. Even if you choose to supplement with a bottle, continue to nurse and/or pump. Your body will make the amount of milk demanded of

it. Continue to demand milk and your body will supply it. Allow the baby to nurse on both sides to optimize your milk production. Buy or rent a good breast pump to allow you to express and store your breast milk.

2. Be sure to continue to take your prenatal vitamins and eat! Your body will demand lots of calories to make milk. This is no time to count calories.

3. Be sure to drink a glass of water with each nursing session.

4. Allow lots of time for rest. Limit visitors, or better yet, ask them to hold the baby so you can nap. Arrange a supplemental feeding schedule at night, where you nurse at 9 p.m. and then you go to bed and sleep until 3 a.m. Allow your partner to bottle-feed pumped breast milk or formula at midnight. This way, you'll both get at least six hours of continuous sleep. (You sleep from 9 p.m. to 3 a.m. and your partner sleeps from 12 midnight to 6 a.m.). This schedule works well for bottle feeders as well. It also allows for the introduction of the bottle, which can help in the future, if you need to supplement or have others feed your child.

5. Be sure to place the baby properly on the breast. Sore nipples are often caused by incorrect placement. The baby's mouth must open fully to take the entire nipple and areola (the brown part), not only the nipple. If the baby just takes the nipple, you will get sore. Stroke the baby's cheek until he/she turns and seems to yawn widely and then quickly place the baby on the breast. You must be fast, or the baby's mouth will close. If this happens, try again.

6. Try to relax. Relaxation allows your milk to let down. Try massaging a few drops of milk from your breast before putting the baby on the nipple. This gets the process started. Sometimes a warm shower helps the milk to let down, or even just the sound of running water can help.

7. Be sure to use your finger to break the suction seal before pulling the baby off the breast. Otherwise…owwww.

8. Do not allow the baby to nurse for hours on end initially and be sure NOT to fall asleep with the baby on your breast. You don't want to fall asleep holding your child as you may drop him/her. Limit your

nursing time to 10 to 15 minutes on each breast, but feed on both breasts if possible. If your nipples are already extremely sore, you can drop the time to 7 to 10 minutes on each breast, but at the end you may want to supplement with a bottle of formula to be sure that the baby isn't still hungry. Remember the goal is a healthy baby.

9. Many breast-feeding advocates do not recommend any bottle feeding until after breastfeeding has been firmly established, usually by four to six weeks. You should read the literature and come to a decision based on your comfort level. I tell my patients that my objective is always the health and safety of the infant. There are times that I do use a bottle of formula (alternative options: tube or syringe feed) with a breast-fed infant, especially if the baby has weight loss. Please consult your provider for specific situations.

10. If you know that you'll be returning to work, as I did, then you know that you'll need to be doing some bottle supplementation with either pumped breast milk or formula. If you introduce a bottle, even just once daily, before the age of six weeks, then the baby should be more comfortable accepting the bottle while you are at work.

11. Working moms do have a right to have a clean, private space, and reasonable unpaid breaks to express milk during work hours without experiencing discrimination, thanks to the Breastfeeding Promotion Act of 2011.

Do I need to give vitamin supplements to my baby if I breastfeed?

We need to discuss what breast milk is lacking: specifically, some vitamins and iron. Breast milk is lacking in vitamin D and iron. Yes, I know you are taking your vitamins, but since we are seeing an increase in breastfeeding, we are also seeing increases in certain disorders of nutrition, such as rickets, a bone disorder caused by a deficiency in vitamin D. Vitamin D is added to our milk, it is added to formula, but is not in adequate supply in breast milk. Your body can produce small amounts of vitamin D by itself, when the skin has sunlight exposure. Babies also need a great amount of iron, as it is not well absorbed by the body. Babies can get iron in iron fortified cereal and in table meat. Baby food jar meats have little iron. Iron is important to prevent anemia.

The AAP recommends, for breastfed infants, vitamin D supplementation starting in the first few days of life, and then iron supplementation starting at four months. The previous recommendation of vitamin D alone has been replaced with the Poly-Vi-Sol with iron. Some providers prefer to start D-vi-sol initially and change to Poly-vi-sol with iron at four months, however, this can be confusing to some parents. It is acceptable to start a vitamin supplement called Poly-Vi-Sol with Iron within the first few weeks if you are breastfeeding.

As taste can be an issue with any iron, there is now a great tasting NovaFerrum Multivitamin with iron drops which can be used in lieu of the Poly-Vi-Sol with iron. These naturally sweetened raspberry-grape flavored vitamin drops are Kosher and vegan verified. They contain no alcohol, dye, lactose, gluten, peanuts, tree nuts, corn, dairy, or soy. These over-the-counter supplements can be purchased at a grocery or drug store.

Iron is essential to all infants. Breast-fed babies will need additional vitamins with iron. Formula-fed infants do not need the additional vitamins with iron, as the iron is added to the formula. Iron can change the color of the infant's stool to black. It can also firm the stools somewhat. You may remember that your prenatal vitamins caused black stools and may have caused some constipation for you. We will discuss constipation further in Chapter 8, but you may consider the addition of apple, prune or pear juice two to four ounces daily, which will soften firm stools in a baby. Most babies do not need daily juice.

How long should you breastfeed?

The choice to continue or stop breastfeeding is entirely up to you, your baby, and your individual situation. Some mothers are only able to nurse for a few weeks before they return to work but may continue to nurse in the morning and evening. Some find that they are not able to produce enough milk to satisfy a particularly ravenous youth. This was my situation. They may supplement with formula yet continue to nurse as well at each feed. I generally recommend 10 to 15 minutes of nursing, followed by supplemental formula in these cases.

Important Tip: Bottle Supplementation

If you wish to supplement your breastfeeding with a bottle, I recommend starting to offer the bottle once daily, starting generally no later than six weeks of life. You can offer either pumped breast milk or formula. By giving one daily bottle, this becomes normal for the baby. Otherwise, a breast-fed infant may struggle to accept a bottle, leading to some difficulty when you want a day off to run a few errands, or if you decide to return to work.

Whatever you decide, you know that you have given your baby your breast milk, passing along those initial antibodies which help protect your baby from common illnesses. We also know that breast-fed infants tend to have fewer ear infections. There is even some recent information which suggests that breast-fed infants are at a lower risk for later obesity. You have done your best to provide your baby with your breast milk.

Some mothers desire to wean from the breast around 12 to 18 months of age, yet others decide to continue breastfeeding until the age of two or three years. There are no rules; you must decide what is right for you and your baby.

What if your body simply is not making enough milk, if you need return to work, or you just are not enjoying the experience?

Formula feeding

There can be so much pressure to breastfeed, and so much guilt is placed on mothers to do so. There are many reasons why a mother may choose not to breastfeed. You may have felt like I did after my first delivery: sick, tired, and needing to return to work. You may not enjoy the experience, as it is uncomfortable at first. You may be like I was while nursing my daughter, and you just don't make enough breast milk to satisfy a very hungry infant. You may have health concerns. Please do not allow anyone's comments or their judgment to interfere with what is best for you and your child. There is no law that says you must breastfeed. You are not a bad mother for choosing a safe, healthy alternative way to feed your baby. If you feel your healthcare providers are discriminating against you for formula feeding, perhaps you should seek alternative care. Some healthcare facilities will not offer formula, and then require that you request it if you desire formula. If you desire formula, simply say so. There is no shame in this option. I would rather a parent be honest with me. Believe me, I can understand both sides of this discussion. Formula is safe and nutritious. There are cases where as a healthcare provider I do recommend formula for the health and safety of the infant, especially if the infant has poor weight gain during attempts to breastfeed.

Today we have many safe and nutritious options. There are numerous formulas available. Babies can and will thrive on infant formula. I do NOT recommend things like goat's milk, cow's milk, or carnation sweetened milk. Nutritionally these are lacking in critical nutrients growing babies need, and these can be harmful or deadly to infants.

Formula Choices

Today we have LOTS of safe and healthy choices. They fall into three main categories:

- Milk-based formulas
- Soy-based formulas
- Specialty formulas

How to Choose a Formula

1. It is generally recommended to begin with one of the milk-based formulas. Most babies do very well on milk-based formula. Be sure to use a formula WITH iron. Low(er)-iron formulas are available but are NOT recommended due to the high demand babies have for iron in their diets. Be sure that when you do a trial of formula, you

continue using that formula for five to seven days before judging the results. Why? It takes three to four days for food substances to pass through the body, so we want to be sure to allow time for any other foods to have left the body before evaluating how well this formula is working. Remember it is not unusual for a baby to have a change in stool when formulas are being changed. The stool will also change if a baby transitions from breast milk to formula. This generally resolves with time. There are now milk-based formulas called "sensitive formulas," which are partially digested, making them more tolerable for infant's sensitive tummies. You can ask your healthcare provider if a partially hydrolyzed or "sensitive" formula may be right for your child.

2. Store brand infant formulas are less expensive alternatives to brand name formulas. They are safe to use since they must maintain the same standards as the brand name formulas. They offer complete nutrition for your baby at nearly half the cost of brand name formula. It is better to use a store brand formula than to have to stretch a brand name formula by diluting it. It is not recommended to dilute a formula with extra water to "make it last," but sadly, many people try

to do just that to save money. Diluted formula can compromise your baby's weight gain and his/her health and may even cause seizure. Better to use the less expensive store brand and have enough formula to feed your child. I understand the need to economize, so do it safely by purchasing a store brand formula.

3. Consult your healthcare provider if:
   a. the baby gets a skin rash after introduction of the formula
   b. the baby seems fussy or "colicky" more than four hours/day
   c. the baby has excessive spitting/vomiting despite good burps
   d. the baby has bloody diarrhea

4. Your provider at some point may recommend a trial of a specialty formula. This is something you should discuss with your healthcare provider before trying. Again, be sure that you give the trial five to seven days before evaluating results. Many healthcare providers are skipping the soy formula option, as many babies who do not tolerate milk protein also may not tolerate soy protein. Rest assured that even if your baby does not tolerate milk or soy protein, they will likely be

able to consume milk and soy products after 12 months of age without any problems.

5. If your child continues to experience vomiting, extreme fussiness, colicky abdominal pain, and gas, your healthcare provider may recommend a trial of a specialty formula. These are hypoallergenic formulas. They are not usually needed and are a bit more expensive, however, in persistently difficult cases, they can really help. I recommend you discuss any symptoms with your healthcare provider before trying such a specialty formula. There are also formulas which contain probiotics that may help with sad baby tummies.

6. Is spitting up an issue? Most babies will spit up. This is very common. Its medical name is Gastroesophageal Reflux or GER. It's often called reflux, but it's simply heartburn with a bit of vomiting. Positional changes, including keeping the baby upright for about ten minutes after feeding, is often helpful. Infant cereal (baby oatmeal) may be introduced to help with reflux, but generally should not be started until four months. (Your healthcare provider may recommend it sooner.) Most babies outgrow reflux symptoms by 6 to 12 months.

If your baby is generally happy, occasionally spits up, has no history of cough or pneumonia, and has acceptable weight gain, he/she is what we call a "happy spitter." I always recommend you speak with your healthcare provider, but a happy spitter will likely require no medical treatment. Sometimes less is more. Perhaps your healthcare provider will recommend an antacid (Zantac) to decrease the heartburn pain, but it may not decrease the spitting up. Sometimes I will recommend the addition of an infant probiotic. Consult your pediatric healthcare provider with questions.

Important Tip: Formula or Breast until 12 months

It is crucial to provide breast milk or formula until 12 months of age. Remember if you are breastfeeding, it is also important to give the baby vitamins daily.

How do I transition from the breast or bottle to a cup?

When weaning the infant, begin to offer a cup at mealtimes. I usually recommend the introduction of the cup between 9 and 12 months. Prior to 12 months, the infant should continue to receive breast milk or formula in the cup. One of my physician partners recommends using a cup for both formula (or breast milk) and water (or juice) so that the baby doesn't make a specific association of a beverage to the cup. After 12 months, whole milk (cow's milk) is recommended. Gradually decrease your nursing or bottle-feeding sessions by one session a day weekly. In other words, the first week, offer a cup at breakfast and drop the first a.m. nursing or bottle. The second week offer a cup at breakfast and at lunch, instead of nursing or bottle. Continue gradually decreasing nursing or bottle sessions until the bedtime session is left. Never stop the cuddling or loving! Continue to rock, sing to, and stroke the baby. Again, it is truly your decision, a personal decision, about when to stop breastfeeding. It is yours to make when you are ready. Don't feel pressured by society to discontinue nursing before you and your child are ready to do so.

Solid foods

When do you start foods? I am frequently asked this question in the office. The simple answer is between four and six months. Babies seem to have windows of opportunity for learning things. They learn to eat after four months of age, and before six months of age. It is important to take advantage of that window of time for teaching eating skills.

Whether you are breast or formula feeding, you may begin baby cereals and foods at four months. The first food can be anything you choose except for honey (infants less than one year of age may NOT consume honey due to the risk of botulism). In the past, rice cereal was generally recommended as the first food, mixed with formula or breast milk, and followed by stage 1 baby foods. The current trend is now to recommend single grain infant oatmeal mixed with breast milk or formula, as the first food.

As of late, there has been discussion that it does not matter whether you introduce fruits or vegetables first, but that you begin the feeding process. Use the stage one fruits and vegetables to begin. Around four months of age, you will notice increased drooling as the baby makes saliva and prepares to begin the digestion process. Most experts agree that baby foods should be introduced sometime between four to six months of age. You do not have to wait for the baby to get teeth to start foods. Signs that a baby may be ready to eat solids are the doubling of birth weight, the ability to sit up in a high chair, and a tongue extrusion reflex (baby can stick out their tongue).

Foods should be started before six months of age to catch the window of opportunity when they can learn about eating. Waiting after six months can lead to feeding aversion, when a baby will not take food from a spoon.

If you decide to start with a baby cereal, such as iron-fortified baby oatmeal, you mix about one tbsp. of cereal with about two tbsp. of iron fortified formula or breast milk. It should be soupy. Spoon feed your infant. You can make your own baby food by cooking and blending fresh fruits, vegetables and meats. Do not add salts or flavoring. I recommend avoiding things like canned vegetables for use in baby foods, as they contain a great deal of sodium that babies do not need. Jar baby meats contain very little iron, so table meats can be pureed. Be careful about food preparation safety, as infants can get botulism from incorrectly prepared foods; that can be toxic. You can freeze the food in ice trays and pop a square out one at a time to microwave. Homemade food is wonderful if you have the time to do so. If not, jar baby food is safe and convenient. My youngest would not eat jar food, only homemade. She's still a picky eater to this day! My son loved store bought, previously prepared, jar baby food. You may want to consider starting with a vegetable, then alternating with a fruit. Most babies will enjoy the sweetness of fruits more than the taste of vegetables. It's okay to keep offering them various foods as they are learning about taste, texture, and even temperature of foods. Peaches are cold and slimy but sweet. Green beans are stringy and warm.

You will soon see that eating food is different from drinking from a bottle or breast. Sucking is an instinct. Eating must be learned, and YOU are the teacher! When you first begin spoon feeding your child, he/she will push out everything you push in! This is normal. It's an exploratory process of learning how to move food around with the tongue and how to coordinate chewing and swallowing. Just because your baby makes a face, that doesn't mean that he/she doesn't like the food. They're just not familiar with it yet. It may take several exposures to a food for the child to appreciate and accept it. Keep giving the food to them, to allow them to develop a taste for it. This is part of the learning they need to experience. Your encouragement will go a long way. Plan to work in 5 to 10-minute sessions twice a day to begin.

I recommend feeding infants with a spoon, so they can learn how to move the food around and swallow it. I often see parents take the short cut of placing cereal or food in a bottle. This is not recommended, as it does not teach the techniques of eating that the child needs to learn. Remember, it is not the calories we are trying to shove down, it is the process of eating that we are teaching. It is interesting that a baby learns to eat and learns to speak around the same time. The exercise of moving food with the tongue encourages the different noises a baby can make and helps them learn both to eat and later speak.

As you introduce new foods between the ages of four to six months, you may add one new food every five days. Some parents find it easier to remember this as once weekly. This allows us to identify if your child has an allergy to a certain food. Start with two meals/day initially and then after about two months, increase to three meals/day. This is a great time to get into the habit of a family meal at night. Studies show that children who eat meals at the dinner table (with the TV off) with their families are better adjusted, have fewer weight problems, and are at a lower risk for depression. This is due to the discussion that occurs during meal time. At our house, we review the day by playing high/low. We each give the best part of our day (the high) and the worst part of our day (the low). It helps everyone to understand the joys and trials of others in their family. It also slows the meal, allowing time to get full, so we don't overeat. This is an important social habit to develop. It provides structure for the child's eating and for our own.

As you start to introduce baby foods between four to six months, adding one new food every five days, you may then progress to stage II foods between six to nine months. Each stage is a bit thicker. I usually recommend the addition of stage III foods starting at nine months, along with certain table foods. Continue using iron-fortified baby cereals daily until at least age nine months, or until the baby can eat table meats.

Important Tip: No Honey

Honey must NOT be introduced until AFTER 12 months of age due to the risk of botulism. Honey is the only "forbidden" food unless you have a family history of food allergies or your child has moderate to severe eczema (if so, see next section).

Peanut introduction

Many parents are not aware of the newest guidelines recommending peanut protein introduction to infants. These recommendations are a result of the

LEAP (Learning Early about Peanut Allergy) study in 2015. This study demonstrated that infants who were exposed to peanut protein early had a significant reduction (up to 86%) in the development of peanut allergy. If your child is at low risk for food allergies (no past medical history or family history of food allergies, no past medical history of moderate to severe eczema), then it is **recommended** that you introduce peanut butter at six months of age, giving a small amount at least three times per week. This is easily done by mixing two teaspoons of peanut butter with two teaspoons of warm water (allow to cool before serving). This peanut butter and water mixture can also be added to oatmeal for a delicious treat. You can stir in two tsp of powdered peanut butter into any baby food as well: peanut butter and baby bananas sound delicious. There is also a product called Bamba, which is a peanut containing puff that melts and is easy for babies to consume. 21 pieces of Bamba is a recommended serving. A peanut powder, PB2, can be mixed with water or added to foods. Obviously, these products and peanut butter have less risk of choking than peanuts, which is why they are recommended for infants. Whole peanuts should NOT be given to children less than three years old due to choking risks. Older infants who can feed themselves can enjoy homemade teething biscuits made with peanut butter. You can find recipes at www.NationalPeanutBoard.org. Get more facts at www.PeanutAllergyFacts.org.

If you DO have a family history of food allergies or if your child has moderate to severe eczema, then ask your pediatric healthcare provider for a referral to a pediatric allergist for further testing and recommendations as to if and when you can introduce peanut containing foods to your baby. Do not introduce foods which contain peanut without being under the supervision of a pediatric allergist if you have a family history of food allergies or if your child has moderate to severe eczema.

Whole milk

By 12 months, you will have switched to all table foods and are ready to transition to whole milk. Children should be on formula or breast milk until 12 months of age, and then whole milk from 12 months of age until age two years. If there is a family history of obesity, cardiovascular disease, or dyslipidemia (high cholesterol or fats in the blood) and the child is not underweight, reduced-fat milk is recommended after 12 months. After age two years, skim, 1% or 2% milk is fine. Some babies transition easily…hand them a bottle or cup of milk and we're done. My son transitioned to whole milk like he drank it every day. No problem! Others tend to be pickier, so a gradual transition from full strength formula, to ¾ formula and ¼ whole milk for one week, then ½ formula and ½ whole milk for the second week, then mostly whole milk with just a touch of formula, and finally to whole milk. My daughter was difficult to transition and didn't want to give up her bottle or her formula. Continue to limit juices to no more than two to four ounces each day, however; children really don't need juice. They can eat the fruits instead of drinking the juice.

Introducing a cup

Babies should be introduced to a cup between 9 and 12 months of age. They should be off the bottle by 15 months of age. Nine months of age is a great time to discontinue pacifier use as well. Most babies will give up the "passie" easily at nine months. If you wait, it can become more difficult to discourage. Prolonged pacifier use can affect the dental alignment and may impact speaking.

Do we need follow-up formula?

Follow-up formula is sold and marketed for babies aged 9 to 24 months. It is not generally needed or recommended. Babies younger than one year of age need formula or breast milk. It is recommended to transition to whole milk at a year of age. I will occasionally use the follow-up formula for a particularly thin child, who is not tolerating whole milk well. Although the follow-up formula is generally unnecessary and more expensive, it is certainly not harmful.

Do babies need water?

Every time you give your baby formula or breast milk, you are giving them plenty of fluids, so infants do not need additional water. Water is unnecessary and may be harmful (it may cause seizures) to infants less than six months of age. I do not recommend giving your baby water. Water can be introduced in small amounts (one to two ounces) once daily after six months of age. After a year of age, they can have water more regularly.

Choking

Often babies will gag or choke when learning to eat solid foods. It is important to be prepared for this, and to know what to do when this happens. I always recommend that all parents, grandparents, and baby sitters become certified in infant and child CPR.

These courses teach you what to do in choking situations. You can obtain certification at your local American Red Cross or American Heart Association. This will prepare you for a true choking emergency.

Both of my children choked right in front of me. With my son, he was in a stroller, and I had handed him a hot dog. This was a rookie mistake. Of course, he bit a piece which was too large and choked. In panic, I yelled for help. A crowd gathered (we were at a mall), but no one offered to help or even dial 911. Thankfully, I was properly trained in CPR and knew what to do. After I got the hot dog out of his airway, he screamed at me. Clearly a child in a stroller should not hold a whole hotdog. Lesson learned. You can receive training in infant and child CPR through the American Red Cross or American Heart Association. Contact your local chapter for class information.

My daughter choked in the car, in her car seat on a piece of candy. Always cut up choking foods and do not feed children in strollers or in the car. Children need you to be watching them eat, so that if they do choke you can assist them. Please learn from my mistakes.

CPR training will help you to differentiate an emergency choking episode from some gagging with a coughing spell. A true choking child cannot make noise or take a full breath. If a child is actively coughing, they are not choking. If they are coughing, continue to encourage them to cough. If you get upset, so will your child. Your best bet is to know what to do. Certification in child CPR is one the best gifts you can give your child!

This chapter has explained the basics of feeding and burping your baby. Please follow up with your pediatric healthcare provider for specific questions or concerns you may have about your child. Next…onto diaper duty!

Key points:

- Breast is best.
- Breastfed infants need baby vitamins (Poly-Vi-Sol with Iron).
- NovaFerrum multivitamin with Iron may be used in lieu of Poly-Vi-Sol if taste is an issue.
- Formula provides complete and balanced nutrition.
- Formula fed infants do not need baby vitamins.
- Newborns should be back to their birth weight by two weeks of age.
- Never shake a baby.
- Introduce a daily bottle prior to six weeks of age in breast-fed babies.
- Begin solid foods before age six months of age.
- Honey should not be given before 12 months of age.
- Continue breastfeeding or formula until 12 months of age.
- CPR training can be received from the American Red Cross or the American Heart Association.

Raising Today's Baby

Chapter 8: Diaper duty

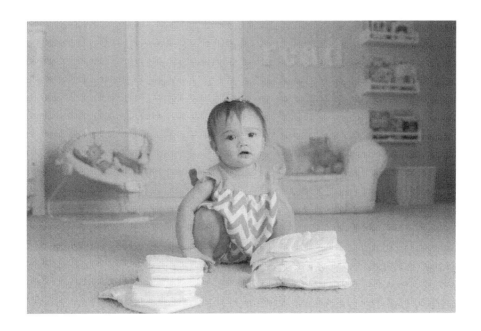

Raising Today's Baby

Chapter 8: Diaper duty

I never thought I'd ever be writing a chapter on baby poo-poo…but here we are because you, the new parent, are going to have MANY concerns about your child's stool. How do I know? Well because I hear it every day in the office. "My baby goes four times a day, or six times a day or once a week," or, "It's green, black, yellow, seedy," followed by, "Is that normal?" Don't worry. That's what we're going to talk about here.

The significance of bowel movements

As a new mom, I was amazed at my level of concern for this topic, which might have disgusted me previously. I was worried when my newborn stooled six times a day, and I was worried when my three-month-old didn't stool for five days. Both, I learned, are normal. I found out it's not necessarily how often they go, but what the stool looks like which is important.

When I became a Certified Pediatric Nurse Practitioner, I quickly discovered that it wasn't just me. All parents seem very concerned with their child's stool. Bowel movements can indicate health or problems both in infants and adults. Sometimes these problems are minor and there is a simple fix, they just pass (catch the pun?) on their own, but other times the problem is serious and requires medical intervention. Parents are concerned about their infant's bowel movements since the infant cannot speak and tell the parent what is wrong. Parents watch the bowel movements as a sign to reassure them of the infant's normality, or they become concerned about potential problems. We want everything to go (again, I jest) smoothly for our perfect little babies, and so we obsessively watch them for signs.

Infant stools can be just as different as individuals are. They vary between children, and at various ages. Eating different foods can change the color and consistency of stools, as can medication or even formula changes. Different doesn't always mean trouble. Different may be a variation of normal. If you are worried, ask your healthcare provider.

Poo facts:

- Newborns generally pass the first stool within the first 24 hours of life. (If your child does not, please tell your healthcare provider.) The first stool is black and tar-like. It is called meconium. Observing your newborn's frequent stooling is one way to confirm that your infant is getting plenty to drink.

- Young babies (prior to one month of age) will generally stool several times a day, even as much as after every feed. The stools are pasty or watery, mushy and occasionally seedy. They vary in color and consistency, and may be mustard colored, black, green, or brown. They often look quite loose.

- Breast-fed infants initially have more and looser stools than formula-fed infants. After two months, breast-fed infants may stool less often than formula-fed infants.

- Around one to two months of age, the stooling patterns change for both breast-fed and bottle-fed infants. Babies then tend to stool much less frequently, perhaps once every few days.

- Breast-fed babies may be even more extreme in their stool changes around two months of age. Some breast-fed babies will make a change from seven or eight daily stools to one stool every five days.

Some will go only once a week. This is not unusual if your child is acting normally. It is not the frequency of the stooling pattern that is concerning, but rather the appearance of the stool itself. It should become larger, more formed, but schmooshable…like Play-Doh. I have many parents who are concerned that their baby is constipated, when in fact, the baby is just having normal bowel movements. Hard, small pellets are not normal and indicate constipation.

- Stools may be all sorts of colors (yellow, brown, green). Any color can be normal except pure white, pure black, and blood-red. Seek medical care if you have concerns about the color of your child's stool.

What if my baby has constipation or diarrhea?

How do you feel if you haven't had a normal bowel movement in a few days? Bloated? Sluggish? Uncomfortable? (Maybe I've been watching too many commercials for fiber additives.) Then, consider how you feel if you've had a few bouts of diarrhea. You may feel fatigued or weak. If our bodies tell us when something is wrong, how much more should we watch our precious children for signs of distress? If you are concerned about your baby's stooling pattern, always consult your healthcare provider.

Constipation

Small hard pellets may be a sign of constipation. However, many parents confuse constipation with normal stools. Remember, it's the consistency, not the frequency. Are the stools formed but soft (like Play-Doh)? If so, it's NOT constipation.

Constipation can be an issue. As stated earlier, formula contains iron. Iron, although very necessary, can have side effects including stomach upset, solid stools, or even diarrhea. Still, iron is VERY necessary. Some parents make the mistake of switching to a low-iron formula in an attempt to help this problem. This is NOT recommended, since you might be creating a second problem...anemia, which is a condition of not enough iron!

Constipation can often be resolved easily enough with the simple addition of juice. This is safe and all natural (even for young babies) and can be given in small amounts (one or two ounces) once or twice daily until stool consistency improves. This will soften most hard stools. When the stools improve, you can discontinue the use of the juice. You can increase their fresh fruit and vegetables, which will help. Baby prunes can be helpful. Apple, prune, and pear juices can loosen stools, and are not harmful to infants in small amounts, such as two to four ounces daily. Your healthcare provider may recommend a prescription fiber additive or infant glycerin suppository. Always seek professional medical advice from your provider before beginning any medication or fiber. When starting a baby on solid foods, you may notice that there are new constipation problems. Adding in a jar or a half a jar of baby prunes is a safe, effective, natural way to defeat this issue.

If your child seems to be in pain or has long bouts of crying associated with a lack of stool, consult your healthcare provider immediately. There are certain health conditions that cause blockages in the bowel which would require immediate medical intervention, especially when accompanied by poor feeding or forceful vomiting.

Diarrhea

Often breast-fed infant's stools are confused with diarrhea since they tend to be seedy and watery. However, infants can also get diarrhea. Diarrhea is loose and watery stools. It may be foul-smelling and is often caused by a virus. One of the particularly dangerous diarrhea-type illnesses seen in infants, Rotavirus, can be prevented with an oral vaccination. It is given in two or three doses at two, four, and sometimes six months of age. It is an important way to prevent diarrhea, which can be life-threatening to a young infant.

The reason diarrhea is so dangerous for babies, especially very young babies, is that they can easily become dehydrated. In serious cases, this dehydration can lead to death if not treated in a timely and appropriate manner. This can be more of an issue in developing countries, where medical care is less available. In developed countries, these infants are usually treated properly and rehydrated, either with oral solutions (fluids) or with IV fluids in an emergency room.

Please seek medical care if you notice blood or mucous in the stools, especially if you've been traveling out of the country, or if the infant shows signs of dehydration (see below). If you have questions, please consult a healthcare provider and don't forget to take a sample of the stool with you for testing.

Signs of dehydration in an infant:

- Lack of tears
- Weakness/lethargy
- Decreased urination: no urine for more than six hours
- Dry, cracked lips
- Sunken fontanel (soft spot)
- Poor feeding
- Weight loss

If you see signs of dehydration, seek immediate emergency medical care at a local hospital or medical clinic.

Antibiotics and diarrhea

Babies who are on antibiotics, such as those given for ear infections, can get diarrhea, which is a normal side effect. Probiotics (the good bacteria that is in yogurt) are helpful. You can find probiotics at your local pharmacy, and this can be sprinkled on the baby's food. Many formulas now also contain probiotics. If your child's formula contains probiotics, then additional probiotics are not necessary. If the diarrhea is excessive after an antibiotic, or there is blood in the stool, contact your healthcare provider immediately. This could be a more serious condition.

Probiotics

There has been great information about the beneficial effects from probiotics. I take a probiotic daily, and give them to my children, now young adults, as well. They provide healthy bacteria for the gut and are thought to offer protective benefits to overall health. I recommend them to my patients.

Diet and diarrhea

Infants with diarrhea should eat a regular diet, but there are foods to avoid and foods to include. Avoid foods which generally loosen stools, such as apple, pear, and prune juice. There are some foods which may help babies have more formed stools. These include bananas, rice, applesauce, and bread products. The child's diet should not be limited to only those foods, but they should have a normal diet which may include those foods. If a child is fed only the BRAT (see below) foods, they may be missing vitamin A, vitamin B12, and calcium, so a varied diet is important.

BRAT diet:

- B for bananas
- R for rice
- A for applesauce (not apple juice)
- T for toast

Even babies as young as four to six months can eat a jar of baby food bananas, if they have been previously introduced. This can help to form stools. Remember from Chapter 7 that it is not recommended to begin feeding babies solid foods prior to four months of age. Beginning solid foods too early can lead to food allergies, and perhaps even obesity. If a baby has diarrhea, this may not be a good time to introduce a new food, so stick to foods which they have already tolerated.

Breast-fed infants should be given a daily baby vitamin with iron, Poly-Vi-Sol with Iron. Formula-fed infants do not need additional vitamin supplements. Sometimes these supplements help stools to become less watery. Sometimes they may aggravate diarrhea or have some minor stomach upset. Always check with your pediatric healthcare provider before beginning any vitamins or medication.

Should I use disposable or cloth diapers?

There are many different types of diapers on the market including disposable and cloth. Cloth may seem friendlier to the environment, but you must consider the entire environmental impact, including water use and electricity use in cleaning the cloth diapers. Most cloth users soak the diapers in bleach water for a time and launder in hot water. There are also diaper services which will pick up and deliver clean disinfected cloth diapers. Cloth has come a long way and now can be purchased with snaps or Velcro, so that you no longer need to use diaper pins.

Disposable diapers are more expensive overall but are more convenient. There is some argument that babies have less diaper rash with disposable diapers, since they are more absorbent than cloth. Although that is something to consider, what really helps prevent diaper rash is frequent changing. If you are trying to save money by not changing a baby frequently, then a child can as easily get a rash in the disposable diapers.

The choice to use cloth or disposable is yours. I have used both. I used cloth with my son to save money, which turned out to be a more time-consuming choice than using disposables. I used disposable diapers with my second child, my daughter, as I was working and much busier, with two young children. I would encourage you to weigh your options and make a choice that works for you and your child. There are situations in which the convenience trumps cost, however, you also may want to consider the environmental cost over personal convenience.

Diaper rash

What do you do when your baby gets that first dreaded diaper rash? Diaper rash is one of life's little problems. It happens. It can be treated and sometimes prevented by good skin care, but at some time it will likely happen. Diaper rash is redness or irritation of the skin within the diaper area. It occurs because of skin breakdown, due to urine or stool. To prevent diaper rash, it is best to keep the skin clean and dry, which can be difficult to do.

Overzealous cleaning can cause irritation instead of preventing it, so I give you a few tips:

1. Only use diaper wipes if the baby has made a stool. If it's just a wet diaper, just take it off, clean the area with a cloth and some warm water, and put a clean diaper on. You don't bathe every time you urinate. If you are routinely bathing your baby, then using a diaper wipe only with stools should suffice.

2. If the baby gets a rash, stop using diaper wipes altogether. Use a clean warm wet washcloth to clean the area. If you must use

diaper wipes, consider switching to non-scented wipes. Try not to be over zealous with cleaning as you may further irritate the sensitive skin.

3. If the baby has a rash, be sure to allow some time with the diaper off to allow the area to air dry, say after bath time. This is very helpful in the healing process.

4. Use a diaper cream which prevents moisture from reaching the skin. There are many on the market, but I recommend Vitamin A+D ointment, Vaseline, Butt Paste, or Desitin.

5. If the area becomes raw, then use only diaper creams that contain zinc, such as Butt Paste or Desitin.

6. If the diaper rash is not clearing up within a week's time, make an appointment to see your healthcare provider. Sometimes rashes are yeast based and require a prescription cream. They also can be bacteria based and require an antibacterial cream. Your healthcare provider can differentiate between these rashes for you.

Done with the diaper change

Now that we have concluded this unpleasant but necessary discussion, we can move on to the next chapter. Remember, it is normal to be rather consumed with the health and condition of your wonderful child. Observing your baby's stool is just one way to do so. One must consider their overall behavior, eating habits, sleeping habits, and general mood. These combine to give us a picture of how the infant is growing and developing.

Key points:

- The first stool, meconium, is passed within the first 24 hours of life.
- Young infants and breast-fed infants stool many times per day.
- Breast-fed infants normally have looser stools than formula-fed infants.
- Stool patterns change around two months of age.
- Small, hard pebbles are a sign of constipation.
- Juice may help with constipation.
- Diarrhea is loose, watery stools.
- Infants can get dehydrated with diarrhea, be aware of signs.
- Diaper rash can be prevented by frequent changes and barrier creams.

Chapter 9: Working out working

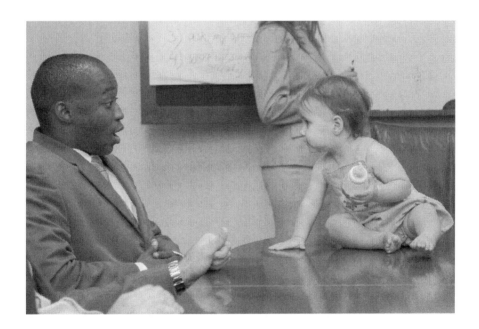

Raising Today's Baby

Chapter 9: Working out working

All parents work, and they work hard. Having a baby and a family is tough work. There's the everyday stuff like meals and laundry. Then, there's the how-do-we-make-ends-meet stuff. For most of us in this economy, there is no decision. We must work outside the home to survive; we must provide for our families. Single parent households fall into this category. For some, there is a priority to work at home and raise their family. This is also a work-related decision, as working at home is still work. Some fathers choose to stay home so their partners can return to work. Finally, some parents face the decision of whether to return to work, work from home, or work as a stay-at-home parent. The truth is that working out working can be tough to do.

I had no choice but to return to work quickly with my first child. Even with my income, we were barely scraping by. I had to return to work, and fast. I barely took four weeks off. With my second child, I had a decision to make, and it was not an easy one. I'm not sure there is a right decision. I feel like I've made them all, and in the end, I found out that finding the balance that is right for your family is the best option.

Deciding to return to work

If you are in the category of having a decision to make about working, don't let anyone pressure you. The choice of whether to go back to work or stay home with your baby is an extremely personal one. I am not here to advocate for one or the other, but rather to present views from both sides to help you find your right fit. I first must admit that I have a personal bias; I am a working mom. I returned to work only one month after delivering my son, which was too soon for me, in my opinion. It was due to necessity, as we were broke. With my daughter, I had more options, and I took the full three months offered, but then shortly after returning to work, decided to be a stay-at-home mom. And then, I'll admit, I survived only six months before taking a job. Some of us just are meant to work on the outside, and others are meant to stay home. There is no greater calling in my humble opinion than that of parent and homemaker. Working as a stay-at-home mom was far more difficult than I ever imagined. Whatever you decide, be sure you go into this decision with your eyes wide open, looking at ALL the factors to help you make a decision that fits you and your family.

Judgment

In a parenting magazine, it was reported that 97% of parents admit that they judge other parents. At first, I found this shocking, but then I realized: who cares? When we stop caring what others think, we are free to do whatever is best for ourselves and our families. Besides, who are they to judge you anyway? Being of a Christian faith, it is not my job to be the judge and jury; we have God for that. Whatever your faith or lifestyle choice, don't feel that you need to live a certain way to please others. Your personal decisions are your own, as are the consequences of those decisions. As you are considering working away from home vs. at home, feel free to do whatever is right for you and your family.

Maternity/paternity leave

First, I would recommend you review your company's policy on maternity/paternity leave. Leave policies vary by company. Most parents end up using a combination of short-term disability, sick leave, vacation days, personal days, and unpaid family leave time. Unfortunately, the United States is the only high-income country without mandatory paid maternity leave for employees. Most states leave it up to the employers to decide whether to provide paid leave. Sweden and Norway have the best parental leave policy in the world and provide more than a year of paid leave for the mother and the father. One of my nurses comes from Sweden and couldn't believe the American leave policy when she had her child in the United States, compared to what was the norm in Sweden. Fortunately, the Family and Medical Leave Act (FMLA) provides that the employee who qualifies can take up to twelve weeks unpaid job protected leave for the birth, adoption, foster care of a child, or to care for a family member with a serious health condition. To qualify, you must have worked for the company for 12 months and served 1,250 hours. Both mothers and fathers can take the leave for a new birth, but the leave must be completed within 12 months. The U. S. armed forces provides 12 weeks of paid leave to the mothers and 10 days of paid leave to the married partner. I would encourage you to take as much maternity/paternity leave as you can afford to. These weeks are precious time with your new infant. You will need the time to rest and recharge, as well as to learn your infant's cycles. When it's time to return to work, you may want to ease your way back in the door. Start with half days or three days a week if you can. Give yourself time to transition back to the "rat race."

Financial burden

You also need to consider the cost and benefit of returning to work. It certainly costs more to have an infant. Just go down the diaper isle at the supermarket and check the prices for diapers and formula. Of course, you have already discovered this fact. Now, consider the additional costs of going to work. Not only will there be child care expenses, but clothing, gas, and dining out is also likely to increase. You may need to hire some help with the housework or gardening. If the cost of child care exceeds what you will be making, choosing the stay-at-home mom option is a no-brainer. After having a child, your pre-baby work clothes may not fit (yet), so you may have to invest in some work attire. Take that into consideration as you make your plans.

Staying at home

You should also consider your personality type. This is something which I clearly did not do. I really wanted to be a stay-at-home mom. I wanted to spend my days interacting with my children, but I found myself bored and broke. I envisioned reading to my child, but she wasn't really interested yet. I wanted to do crafts, but found the days spent on mundane tasks: dishes, laundry, feeding, changing, and wiping children. You know, parenting. My personality did not fit well with staying at home. I have interviewed other parents who felt the same way. I really envy those who thrive within the home environment, but it just wasn't me. First, know thyself. Really examine who you are and who you want to be before making your decision. Never make an important decision when you are tired, hungry, or grouchy.

Next, examine your personal and family needs, as well as the needs of your child. Perhaps you have many children that need your care. Perhaps you have a special needs baby, who would benefit from more home time, allowing for therapies and doctor visits. Perhaps you are a single parent, who needs to return to work as soon as possible to support the family. Perhaps you are a professional, who needs to keep their skills sharp. Maybe you have a partner who travels extensively, and the children would benefit from having a parent at home for stability. Maybe you are a father who wants to be a stay-at-home dad. There are as many possibilities as stars…examine your personal situation and take it into consideration.

Consider the decision of staying home in the context of how you can manage this situation financially without the additional, but needed, income.

Perhaps you can economize by downsizing to one car. Many families do this and use public transportation or share the ride. My parents did this for years, taking each other to work, and waiting to pick the other up. They survived, and even caught an occasional car nap.

Perhaps you can grow a garden to supplement your grocery bill. Some folks have chickens, and always have eggs, a great source of protein. There are shortcuts you can take across the board, such as eating at home rather than dining out. I try to limit dining out to once weekly, and it saves a ton. Couponing is a big fad, but it's also smart. You can really save on your grocery bill this way. Also discount or big-box stores like Costco are a great investment, as you save more, if you buy only what you need. (I've had my share of overspending at Costco.) You can't beat the prices, especially on grocery items.

I find I save money by making a meal plan for a week, then shopping only for those items. It eliminates much of the impulse buy. I also pack lunches for my families, not only saving money, but providing healthy food options for them. Avoid bottled water, a huge rip-off. Instead buy bottles (PBA free) and refrigerate tap water. You can save $1,000 per person per year just by not buying bottled water. Instead of grabbing a daily coffee at Starbucks, make it at home and place it in a travel mug. You can save $1,300/year making your own coffee. We love our Keurig coffee maker, and for the cost of it, you will save a ton at the trendy and expensive coffee spots. How about smoothies at home instead of out? A blender, ice, and fruit and you are set. Homemade pizza is much cheaper (and more delicious) than ordering delivery.

You can let go of the gardener/house keeper, as you will have time to do these things yourself. I do my own cleaning and gardening. I also do my own painting, as painters are very expensive. Let me clarify: when I say I do my own painting, I mean that I decide what I want painted and I buy the paint, and then my husband actually does the work. I supervise and prepare snacks!

Cloth diapers now have snaps and are a cost savings over disposable, and they help the environment. You can also save money by buying previously owned furniture and even some good gently worn clothing. These are just a few cost-saving ideas.

Staying at home activities

If you're thinking about staying at home, consider enrichment activities both for yourself and your child. How will you include socialization and structure to your days? Can you take up some new activities to feel fulfilled, such as painting or gardening? How can your child gain enrichment from other children? Consider play groups or outings. Most local baby-wearers groups meet regularly. There are mom's groups at churches. I think if I would have had better socialization, I might have succeeded as a stay at home mom. Also, consider how any older children may feel about you staying at home. I have a friend who shared that her older child begged to return to daycare, as staying at home with the new baby was "sooooo boring". Consider what kind of routine you want to develop. Mine included sleeping as much as possible and catching up with my morning TV routine (love that GMA). Maybe not the best plan. Babies need structure. They need to wake, eat, play, and nap within a schedule. The more consistent you are with their schedules, the better they do. Some flexibility is good, but scheduling is the key.

Working from home

With the creation of the internet and computer technology, many jobs don't have to take place "in an office setting". Look into the option of working from home. This allows the flexibility of parenting while also working. Consider that you still may need some child care help for important meetings or online discussions. The flexibility of being able to tele-commute eliminates the time needed for commuting in traffic, the need for an expensive wardrobe, and limits the need for child care. Go into such a job with your eyes open, as working from home can be difficult if you are easily distracted. There are always dishes and laundry at home which may distract you from work. You also will need to organize your work schedule around your child's needs.

Special needs children

Our special needs children deserve a special paragraph. As I've recently met a new special needs baby, who I vowed NOT to fall in love with, and then did, I must address this topic. Parents of special needs babies need flexibility and extra time. My editor shared with me that the stresses of parenting a special needs child includes the challenge of trying to hold down a job, while juggling doctor visits, physical therapy visits, and sick days. She stated that after it was clear that her son had serious and chronic medical issues, she decided not to return to publishing right away, but instead opened a home daycare to allow her to be home with her son. Within a year, she forged a work plan to do freelance editorial work from home and built a business that serviced literary agents and authors (such as myself), without having to go into an office. She could work when her child slept: early mornings, late at night, or during naps, as well as over the weekend when her husband was home. She worked from the soccer sideline with a red pen and manuscripts (before the days of Kindles and iPads) and wrote reports and scheduled business calls while her son was in school. When he was hospitalized, which unfortunately happened frequently, she moved into the hospital with him, and then worked on her laptop from his bedside. She didn't have to worry about losing her job due to missed work days. This is an example of real devotion to parenting, and just another reason why I respect my editor so very much. This is a great example of how working from home can work for you.

Professional awareness

Consider your profession as well. I know many physicians and nurses who practice just one or two days a week to keep their licenses up to date but want the flexibility to care for their children. You may want to consider how staying at home will impact your career options in the future. I met a master's degree prepared nurse practitioner who has been out of the workforce for nearly 20 years while raising her children. She wants to get back into her career, but her knowledge base is so outdated that without additional training and re-licensing, it would be nearly impossible. When she was working, hospitals didn't even use computers. Now, everything is done on computers. You may want to consider keeping your hand in the pool of your profession to stay up to date. Again, I acknowledge my professional bias as a working mother, but I know a PhD psychologist who strongly advises women to keep their hands in the career pot. Stepping away can be a setback, if not detrimental to your career. Most companies base their salary offer on your last salary. If your last salary was ten years ago, then you won't be offered the going rate and you won't be up to date on the latest changes.

You will need to consider a job's flexibility. With a new baby, you will see the doctor at least every two to three months during the infant's first year of life. Can you get time off for doctor visits? Will your partner or family member help you with sick days? Does your job allow you the time and place to pump breast milk if you are a nursing mom? Most companies are required to allow you both the time and a place to pump breast milk. Most companies give you sick time, but some frown on using them for your children instead of yourself.

Consider if you can use flex hours to make up lost work time, or even work from home. I know a nursing mom who negotiated a full-time schedule as three and a half days in the office, and the other day and a half at home for administration work. Other jobs offer job sharing. I know of two moms who accepted one full-time job. One works three days one week, while the other works two days and vice versa the next week. They split the income and benefits down the middle. After trying a full-time position with travel, and thoroughly exhausting myself within a year, I opted for a part-time job, three to four days/week, which allowed me the flexibility to care for my children, pursue my doctoral research, teach online at a local university, and write this book. I've been at my position for sixteen years now, and I love every day. Flexibility helps working mothers. You may want to consider a work-at-home option. With the Internet, and availability of faxing, scanning, and emailing, as well as face-time and Skype, there is no reason to have to be somewhere when the computer allows you to work from home. This not only cuts down on commuting time and costs but improves job satisfaction and productivity. It's quite a viable option these days. I teach an online class from time to time with a local university, and I love that it allows me to work in my free time on my own schedule (in comfy clothes). Telecommuting is a growing trend.

Child care

You will need to consider your available resources, such as daycare. You want to look not only at the cost of daycare, but at the convenience and hours as well. Most daycares operate only from 6 a.m. to 6 p.m. Monday to Friday, so if your job requires evenings or weekends, you will need to make other arrangements. My daycare charged five dollars each minute you were late after 6 p.m. picking up your child, so if traffic was bad, I got a penalty. You may want to consider private in-home nannies, private home daycare centers, and state-licensed daycares. There are small options and larger ones. You will have to consider cost, convenience, and safety.

My first concern with hiring a nanny or sitter was that I was afraid that my child would love her more than me. I needn't have worried. You want your child to form an attachment to their care provider, but a child always loves their parents. You also want to consider what enrichment is offered. I hate it when children are plopped in front of the TV. (Sure, I've done it myself, but still hate it.) There is something to be said for the convenience of having a nanny come to your home. You don't have to wake, dress, or feed your child before heading to work. They come to you. The cost is generally higher, and sometimes includes some light housework. It may be ideal if you have several children who need to be picked up and dropped off during the day. Unfortunately, if your nanny is late, so are you. If your nanny is sick, then what? I loved having a nanny come to the house, but I did experience a few unexpected surprises. One day, returning home early and unexpectedly, I found her in my closet trying on my clothes. Odd? Indeed. She was terminated. Another nanny decided to re-arrange the furniture. You can guess about her career path as well.

I decided that the invasion of my personal space was not worth the convenience, so I transitioned my son to a private home daycare. The lady was lovely, and she only cared for a few children at a time. I felt like my son was safe and was in a place where he was loved. She was happy to follow any specific directions I had for her, and she was quite cooperative. Unfortunately, when one kid got sick, so did all the others. I also questioned if my child was getting enough one on one care, as there was some TV time noticed. I did feel like the caregiver cared about my son and that it was a safe and healthy option. I hated having to get him up early, fed and dressed. It sometimes felt like morning was a battle zone under a stop watch. Sadly, the nice lady decided to return to work, and closed her daycare. Next, I tried other home daycare options. One day I picked up my son after work. I was informed that he was "bad" that day, and for punishment he didn't get lunch. I never took him back. Just the thought that withholding food could in any way be an appropriate consequence for poor behavior makes me shiver. How absurd. I was so angry. Of course, I had to call in to work the next day to make other daycare arrangements.

You may wish to consider family members for child care. Although I have heard it recommended that a care giver with a genetic attachment may provide the best care to young children, I personally have concerns about the use of a family member in this manner. It has been my experience that family members may not be adequately compensated, which may lead to bad feelings. Also, not everyone parents in the same manner, so you may not wish for your child to learn unhealthy habits that your family member may teach. Children learn what they live. Also, be sure to stress that family members need to be current on CPR, and safety items such as sleeping on the back, and car seat safety.

As I got older, I got wiser. I toured public daycare facilities and looked at licenses. I considered the ratio of caregivers to children and the cleanliness of the facility. I decided only to use licensed permanent daycare facilities for several reasons. They are a safer option as there is usually more than one caregiver to a room. If you have an issue, you can discuss it with the manager, who then can handle the staff. They have set hours, so if one provider is ill, they call in a back-up. The cost is predetermined and prearranged, so you know what to expect. I ended up using the same daycare for both children for many years. The name you ask…La Petite Academy. Although my experiences were not perfect, they did effectively handle any situations that arose. They provided structure for the children, safety, nutrition, and enrichment. I also learned to have a back-up plan. I had a group of moms who would back up each other for evening meetings,

Saturday events, or the occasional Friday night movie. We traded hours to keep things fair. As a military spouse, I often had to handle situations alone, so this made life much easier. Better to be prepared than not.

Benefits of child care

There's also a social dynamic in daycare that I adore. Children encourage each other to try, to learn, and to grow. This type of socialization is priceless. I remember dropping my child off at daycare after dressing and feeding her. Let me add here that it's important to make drop-off quick to make it less painful. After a particularly tearful drop-off, I waited a minute then peeked through the class window. She was laughing and playing. Kids are resilient, and they do best when you don't drag out the drama. Anyway, when I picked her up, she was clearing and wiping a table. I had no idea that my 18-month-old could even do that! Kids show other kids how to act, how to share, and even how to solve disputes. One time my daughter was bitten, and another time she was the biter. Neither behavior was encouraged, but lessons were learned. She hardly ever bites anyone now that she's an adult, but I'm careful around her the first thing in the morning.

Education is an important part of child care. Most facilities routinely incorporate learning activities into the day. You can be assured that your child isn't watching TV for eight straight hours. They work on numbers, colors, letters, and shapes. They work with sand, water, and bubbles. They encourage developmental and physical skills through use of tricycles and play yards. Children who attend daycare are starting the educational process at a younger age, which may help them to better prepare for advanced education in the future.

Juggling a career with parenthood

Sometimes after a crazy day at work, I am so thankful to get into my car for the drive home. I blare the music and take a mental break to prepare me to face my next job, parenting. It can be rough to walk into the house after a long day and look at the work still to be done. There's picking up from childcare/after school/sports. There's the task of dinner. I do best when I plan dinner in the morning before work. The crock-pot is a working mom or dad's friend. There are homework projects and report cards. There are errands and housework. There is bath time and then clothing preparation. Just thinking of it, I remember sitting in the driveway, just for a minute, to catch my breath before going in.

Raising Today's Baby

The key to calming the chaos is preparation. If I put food in the crock-pot, and set the table before I go to work, then we can all sit right down to dinner. If not, I suggest setting out some carrots and celery to calm the starving beasts as you prepare the meal. Try to keep dinner time simple but sit down together at the table. We have found that families that eat together at the table, with the TV off, tend to have healthier relationships and less problems. It gives everyone time to speak. Don't try to conquer the chaos by yourself. Divide and conquer. I'm a big believer in everyone helping to prepare and clean up. Even a young child can clear the table, push in chairs, and wipe up. Try to have a set schedule and stick to it. Keep the TV off during the week to encourage homework and reading. My kids weren't allowed any TV between Monday and Thursday. There's too much to do each evening, and TV is a time killer as well as a distraction. Kids who read do better at school. Limit bath time. My kids love to swim in the tub. I set a timer in their bathroom, and when the timer went off, time to get out. I usually allowed about 15 minutes (supervised for younger children) for a bath or shower. Set out the clothing for the next day. It really helps your morning. Take a few minutes to read to your children before bed. A book only takes about five to ten minutes to read but makes a huge difference. This is a great time to listen to your children about their concerns. Take some time to organize your evening schedule and your chaos may turn into calm. After you get the kids tucked in at 8:00 or 8:30 p.m., then you can have some private time of your own to relax.

Balance

All in all, you need to find some balance for you and your family. That may include returning to work or staying at home. Some reasons to work include financial pressures, social interaction, professional aspiration, and educational fulfillment. There are different job types, including full-time, part-time, job sharing, or working from home. Some reasons to stay home include bonding with your child, ease of breastfeeding, cost of day care exceeding income, ease of doctor's visits, and special needs children. There is no one right or wrong answer. Find what works for you and your family. I hope that this chapter helps you in your decision-making process, and that you can find peace in your work-life balance.

Key points:

- Working at home or returning to work is a personal decision.
- Investigate your maternity/paternity leave benefits.
- Weigh the cost and benefit of returning to work.
- Consider your personality type, family, and personal needs before deciding to return to work or work from home.
- Discuss economic management for staying at home options.
- Research enrichment activities for both parent and child for staying at home.
- Parents of special needs children need time and flexibility in their schedule.
- Consider your profession and how to stay up-to-date.
- Weigh your job's flexibility for sick child days and doctor visits.
- Review child-care options and visit centers.
- Benefits to daycare include structure, education, and social interaction.
- Juggling a career with parenthood can be done with preparation and organization.
- Find balance in your life in working at home or away from home.

Epilogue

As I close this book, I am pleased that I've had this opportunity to share my insight and some of my life experiences with my readers. This second edition has included recent updates (such as peanut introduction) based on research. I hope that you may learn from my struggles as a mom, and from my work as a pediatric healthcare provider. I also hope that I can make your parenting journey a little less stressful, and a little more joyful. My mission is to help parents raise healthy, happy children.

Watch for my next book: *Raising Today's Toddler*, available soon on Amazon!

Read more at www.RaisingTodaysChild.com

Follow me on Facebook.com/RaisingTodaysChild

and on Twitter.com/Rzn2dayschild

Raising Today's Baby

About the Author

Dr. Melanie J. Wilhelm is a Pediatric Nurse Practitioner in Norfolk, VA, as well as Adjunct Assistant Professor at Old Dominion University. She obtained a Bachelor of Science Degree with honors from Bowling Green State University, Ohio, completed a Master of Science with honors at Old Dominion University, Virginia, and obtained Certification as a Pediatric Nurse Practitioner. She completed the Doctor of Nursing Practice at Old Dominion University with a research focus on pediatric obesity related to nutrition counseling.

Dr. Wilhelm writes a monthly column for the Tidewater Family Magazine. Her research study on pediatric obesity was published in the Infant, Child, and Adolescent Nutrition Journal in October 2012. She has been published several times in the national parenting magazine *Ready, Set, Grow*. Her poster on Pediatric Obesity related to Nutrition Counseling was accepted at the National Institute of Children's Healthcare Quality (NICHQ) annual conference in 2010. She received the 1990 Teacher of the Year Award for the Southern Association of Colleges.

Dr. Wilhelm belongs to the National Association of Pediatric Nurse Practitioners and served as President of the local Hampton Roads Chapter in 2007. She is a member of the American Academy of Pediatrics, the Daughters of the American Revolution, and St. Stephen Martyr Catholic Church. She is married with two adult children and resides in Virginia. Her life mission statement is to help parents raise healthy, happy children.

Visit her website at www.RaisingTodaysChild.com. Follow her on Facebook.com/RaisingTodaysChild and Twitter.com/Rzn2dayschild.

Raising Today's Baby

Dr. Melanie J. Wilhelm DNP CPNP

Doctor of Nursing Practice, Certified Pediatric Nurse Practitioner

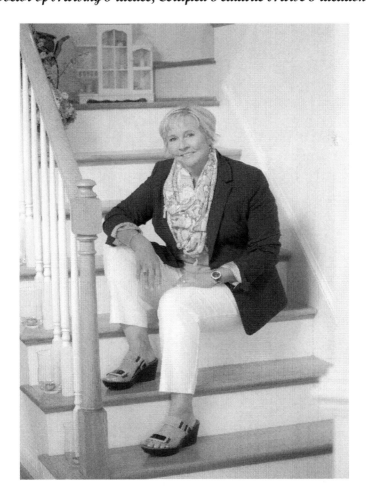

Raising Today's Baby

Made in the USA
Columbia, SC
13 May 2021